Hearing Loss Research at NIOSH

Reviews of Research Programs of the National Institute for Occupational Safety and Health

Committee to Review the NIOSH Hearing Loss Research Program

Board on Health Sciences Policy

INSTITUTE OF MEDICINE AND
NATIONAL RESEARCH COUNCIL
OF THE NATIONAL ACADEMIES

THE NATIONAL ACADEMIES PRESS
Washington, D.C.
www.nap.edu

THE NATIONAL ACADEMIES PRESS   500 Fifth Street, N.W.   Washington, DC 20001

NOTICE: The project that is the subject of this report was approved by the Governing Board of the National Research Council, whose members are drawn from the councils of the National Academy of Sciences, the National Academy of Engineering, and the Institute of Medicine. The members of the committee responsible for the report were chosen for their special competences and with regard for appropriate balance.

This study was requested by the National Institute for Occupational Safety and Health of the Centers for Disease Control and Prevention and supported by Contract Nos. 200-2000-00629 (Task Order #0033) and 200-2005-10881 (Task Order #0004), between the National Academy of Sciences and the Centers for Disease Control and Prevention. Any opinions, findings, conclusions, or recommendations expressed in this publication are those of the author(s) and do not necessarily reflect the view of the organizations or agencies that provided support for this project.

International Standard Book Number-10: 0-309-10274-X
International Standard Book Number-13: 978-0-309-10274-2

Additional copies of this report are available from the National Academies Press, 500 Fifth Street, N.W., Lockbox 285, Washington, DC 20055; (800) 624-6242 or (202) 334-3313 (in the Washington metropolitan area); Internet, http://www.nap.edu.

For more information about the Institute of Medicine, visit the IOM home page at: **www.iom.edu.**

Copyright 2006 by the National Academy of Sciences. All rights reserved.

Printed in the United States of America.

Suggested Citation: Institute of Medicine and National Research Council. 2006. *Hearing Loss Research at NIOSH.* Committee to Review the NIOSH Hearing Loss Research Program. Rpt. No. 1, Reviews of Research Programs of the National Institute for Occupational Safety and Health. Washington, DC: The National Academies Press.

THE NATIONAL ACADEMIES
Advisers to the Nation on Science, Engineering, and Medicine

The **National Academy of Sciences** is a private, nonprofit, self-perpetuating society of distinguished scholars engaged in scientific and engineering research, dedicated to the furtherance of science and technology and to their use for the general welfare. Upon the authority of the charter granted to it by the Congress in 1863, the Academy has a mandate that requires it to advise the federal government on scientific and technical matters. Dr. Ralph J. Cicerone is president of the National Academy of Sciences.

The **National Academy of Engineering** was established in 1964, under the charter of the National Academy of Sciences, as a parallel organization of outstanding engineers. It is autonomous in its administration and in the selection of its members, sharing with the National Academy of Sciences the responsibility for advising the federal government. The National Academy of Engineering also sponsors engineering programs aimed at meeting national needs, encourages education and research, and recognizes the superior achievements of engineers. Dr. Wm. A. Wulf is president of the National Academy of Engineering.

The **Institute of Medicine** was established in 1970 by the National Academy of Sciences to secure the services of eminent members of appropriate professions in the examination of policy matters pertaining to the health of the public. The Institute acts under the responsibility given to the National Academy of Sciences by its congressional charter to be an adviser to the federal government and, upon its own initiative, to identify issues of medical care, research, and education. Dr. Harvey V. Fineberg is president of the Institute of Medicine.

The **National Research Council** was organized by the National Academy of Sciences in 1916 to associate the broad community of science and technology with the Academy's purposes of furthering knowledge and advising the federal government. Functioning in accordance with general policies determined by the Academy, the Council has become the principal operating agency of both the National Academy of Sciences and the National Academy of Engineering in providing services to the government, the public, and the scientific and engineering communities. The Council is administered jointly by both Academies and the Institute of Medicine. Dr. Ralph J. Cicerone and Dr. Wm. A. Wulf are chair and vice chair, respectively, of the National Research Council.

www.national-academies.org

COMMITTEE TO REVIEW THE NIOSH HEARING LOSS RESEARCH PROGRAM

BERNARD D. GOLDSTEIN (*Chair*), Professor, Department of Environmental and Occupational Health, Graduate School of Public Health, University of Pittsburgh, Pennsylvania

BETH A. COOPER, Manager, Acoustical Testing Laboratory, NASA John H. Glenn Research Center at Lewis Field, Cleveland, Ohio

SUSAN E. COZZENS, Professor, School of Public Policy, Georgia Institute of Technology, Atlanta

KAREN J. CRUICKSHANKS, Professor, Department of Population Health Sciences and Department of Ophthalmology and Visual Sciences, University of Wisconsin Medical School, Madison

JUDY R. DUBNO, Professor, Department of Otolaryngology–Head and Neck Surgery, Medical University of South Carolina, Charleston

DENNIS A. GIARDINO, Acoustical Consultant, Pittsburgh, Pennsylvania

RENA H. GLASER, Manager of Medical Surveillance (Retired), 3M Corporation, St. Paul, Minnesota

WILLIAM W. LANG, President, Noise Control Foundation, Poughkeepsie, New York

LAURA C. LEVITON, Senior Program Officer for Research and Evaluation, Robert Wood Johnson Foundation, Princeton, New Jersey

BRENDA L. LONSBURY-MARTIN, Research Professor, Division of Otolaryngology, Department of Surgery, Loma Linda University School of Medicine, Loma Linda, California

MICHAEL A. SILVERSTEIN, Clinical Professor, Department of Environmental and Occupational Health Sciences, School of Public Health and Community Medicine, University of Washington, Seattle

Framework Committee Liaison

FRANKLIN E. MIRER, Director, Health and Safety Department, United Automobile, Aerospace and Agricultural Implement Workers of America (UAW), Detroit, Michigan

Project Staff

LOIS JOELLENBECK, Senior Program Officer
JANE DURCH, Senior Program Officer
KRISTEN GILBERTSON, Research Assistant

Independent Report Reviewers

This report has been reviewed in draft form by individuals chosen for their diverse perspectives and technical expertise, in accordance with procedures approved by the National Research Council's Report Review Committee. The purpose of this independent review is to provide candid and critical comments that will assist the institution in making its published report as sound as possible and to ensure that the report meets institutional standards for objectivity, evidence, and responsiveness to the study charge. The review comments and draft manuscript remain confidential to protect the integrity of the deliberative process. We wish to thank the following individuals for their review of this report:

Kathleen Campbell, Department of Surgery, Southern Illinois University School of Medicine
William W. Clark, Program in Audiology and Communication Sciences, Washington University School of Medicine in St. Louis, Missouri
Christine Dixon-Ernst, Occupational Health Issues and EHS Information Systems, Alcoa, Pittsburgh, Pennsylvania
Joseph A. Main, Consultant, Mining Health and Safety, Spotsylvania, Virginia
Susan Megerson, Intercampus Program in Communicative Disorders, The University of Kansas
David Roessner, School of Public Policy, Georgia Institute of Technology
Kenneth Rosenman, Division of Occupational and Environmental Medicine, Michigan State University

Scott D. Sommerfeldt, Department of Physics and Astronomy, Brigham Young University, Provo, Utah

Evelyn Talbott, Department of Epidemiology, University of Pittsburgh, Pennsylvania

Although the reviewers listed above have provided many constructive comments and suggestions, they were not asked to endorse the conclusions or recommendations nor did they see the final draft of the report before its release. The review of this report was overseen by **Paul D. Stolley**, University of Maryland School of Medicine, and **David G. Hoel**, Medical University of South Carolina. Appointed by the National Research Council and Institute of Medicine, they were responsible for making certain that an independent examination of this report was carried out in accordance with institutional procedures and that all review comments were carefully considered. Responsibility for the final content of this report rests entirely with the authoring committee and the institution.

Preface

It has been a great pleasure to work with the group of consummate professionals who served on the Committee to Review the NIOSH Hearing Loss Research Program. The committee was fortunate that the Institute of Medicine's recognition of the unusual challenges posed by this report led to its assigning particularly superb staff to work with us. The dedication, hard work, and patience of Lois Joellenbeck and Jane Durch were essential to the completion of this task. Kristen Gilbertson's very able assistance deserves high praise as well.

We also want to thank the many individuals working for NIOSH (National Institute for Occupational Safety and Health) with whom we interacted. Being reviewed produces anxiety in any organization—and this is particularly true now that accountability is so prominent in the pronouncements of the Office of Management and Budget and of Congress. The discomfort of NIOSH participants was no doubt exacerbated by our committee's own learning curve, which led to many requests for different types of information, and by the lack of familiarity of NIOSH professionals with this new review process, which was still evolving during their preparation of materials for this committee. We hope that this has been a valuable learning experience both for NIOSH and for future National Academies committees reviewing NIOSH research programs.

Our committee was presented with a number of challenges that went beyond the usual assignment of analyzing and synthesizing information about a program and then making recommendations. No previous committee had worked under this new NIOSH review program, which may include up to 14 other similar reviews in the next few years, so we had no template to follow and were constrained to develop a format that would work not only for us but for future committees. Fortunately, we were provided with very helpful guidance for this new approach, including meeting the challenge of scoring the Hearing Loss Research Program both for impact and for relevance, by the National Academies' Committee for the Review of NIOSH Research Programs (known as the Framework Committee). We greatly appreciated the valuable and patient input of Frank Mirer, the liaison from the Framework Committee; Evan Douple and Sammantha Magsino, the Framework Committee study staff; and David Wegman, the Framework Committee chair. Of particular note is that the scoring system for impact and relevance is in whole numbers and is not linear (i.e., a score of 3 is not equidistant from a 1 and a 5). Determining the scores required careful review of the definitions that were provided to us by the Framework Committee. Conforming to the definitions and outline of the Framework Committee required many iterations.

When the overall review process is completed, scores for impact and relevance will be available for the 15 NIOSH components evaluated. Inevitably, and unfortunately, comparisons among these NIOSH programs are likely to be made based on the score alone. I urge readers to go beyond the scores to read both the commentary that is the basis for the score and the specific committee recommendations.

The need to go beyond the scores for impact and relevance is particularly pertinent for a cross-cutting matrix organization such as the Hearing Loss Research Program. A standard linear logic model of the type on which this review is based begins with inputs, such as funding and staff; moves through outputs, the direct products of the program; and proceeds to outcomes, the extent to which the mission and goals of the organization have been attained. Evaluating whether the NIOSH Hearing Loss Research Program uses its inputs appropriately is complicated by two factors. First, as a classic matrix organization that has its components within various NIOSH line organizations, the Hearing Loss Research Program does not really have its own budget and staff. As such, it is difficult to evaluate whether the program is making appropriate decisions about inputs. This is further complicated by the need to follow congressional budgetary dictates that can distort the relevance score of the program—for example, devotion of more than half of the Hearing Loss Research Program budget to mining is not consonant with the relative extent to which miners represent the American workforce at risk for hearing loss. Comparisons of final scores may lead the very valuable NIOSH cross-cutting matrix organizations to be ranked lower than NIOSH line organizations due to the dictates of the logic model on which the Framework Committee based its guidance.

The outcomes portion of the logic model also presents some difficulty when evaluating a research organization that does not control how its output is used. NIOSH research output is added to the pool of knowledge from which many others may dip, often in unforeseen ways that do not follow the linearity of a logic model. These externalities are addressed in our review but may be lost if the focus is solely on a numerical score.

What follows is the committee's review of the NIOSH Hearing Loss Research Program. It is our hope that the results of this review will help to further build a dynamic research program responsive to protecting the hearing of American workers and will contribute to the challenging task of developing processes to fairly evaluate government health research organizations.

Bernard D. Goldstein
Committee Chair

Contents

SUMMARY 1

1 **INTRODUCTION** 21
   Study Charge and Evaluation Committee, 22
   The NIOSH Hearing Loss Research Program, 24
   Evaluation Approach, 33
   The Committee's Report, 34
   References, 36

2 **EVALUATION OF THE HEARING LOSS RESEARCH PROGRAM** 37
   Hearing Loss Research Program Goals, 38
   External Factors with Broad Effects on the Hearing Loss
      Research Program, 38
   Other Factors Affecting the Hearing Loss Research Program, 42
   Assessment of Relevance, 43
   Overall Evaluation of the Relevance of the Hearing Loss
      Research Program, 70
   Assessment of Impact, 72
   Overall Evaluation of the Impact of the Hearing Loss
      Research Program, 92
   References, 96

3 **IDENTIFYING EMERGING ISSUES AND RESEARCH AREAS IN OCCUPATIONAL HEARING LOSS PREVENTION** 102
   The Hearing Loss Research Program's Process for Identifying Emerging Issues and Research Areas in Occupational Hearing Loss Prevention, 103
   Committee Assessment of the Hearing Loss Research Program's Identification of Emerging Issues and Research Areas in Occupational Hearing Loss Prevention, 108
   Emerging Issues and Research Areas in Occupational Hearing Loss Prevention Identified by the Evaluation Committee, 110
   Conclusion, 113
   References, 113

4 **RECOMMENDATIONS FOR PROGRAM IMPROVEMENT** 115
   Program Management in a Matrix Environment, 115
   Access to Intramural and Extramural Expertise, 117
   Program Planning, 118
   Evaluation of Hearing Loss Prevention Measures, 120
   Surveillance Activities, 120
   Noise Control Perspective, 121
   Extramural Research, 122
   References, 123

APPENDIXES

A Framework for the Review of Research Programs of the National Institute for Occupational Safety and Health 125
B Methods Section: Committee Information Gathering 168
C Information Provided by the NIOSH Hearing Loss Research Program 186
D Biographical Sketches of Committee Members 197

Tables, Figures, and Boxes

TABLES

1-1 NIOSH Hearing Loss Research Program Funding by Fiscal Year, 1997–2005, 31

2-1 Research Goals and Subgoals of the NIOSH Hearing Loss Research Program, as of February 2006, 40

2-2 NIOSH Hearing Loss Research Program Budget and Staffing by Research Goals, 46

FIGURES

1-1 NIOSH organization chart, as of December 2005, 27
1-2 Location of Hearing Loss Research Program activities in NIOSH, 28
1-3 Logic model for the Hearing Loss Research Program, 35

BOXES

S-1 Scale for Rating Program Relevance, 8
S-2 Scale for Rating Program Impact, 11
S-3 Summary of Recommendations, 20

2-1 Logic Model Terms and Examples, 39
2-2 Scale for Rating Program Relevance, 73
2-3 Scale for Rating Program Impact, 95

3-1 Participants in the NIOSH Hearing Loss Prevention Futures Workshop, 104
3-2 Emerging Research Issues Identified by the Hearing Loss Research Program, 105
3-3 Hearing Loss Prevention Goals in the NIOSH Mining Research Plan, 107

B-1 Agendas for Site Visits, 170
B-2 Letter Inviting Comment on the NIOSH Hearing Loss Research Program, 174
B-3 Emerging Research Areas in Occupational Hearing Loss and Noise Control Suggested by Stakeholders, 176

Abbreviations and Acronyms

AAA	American Academy of Audiology
AAOHNS	American Academy of Otolaryngology–Head and Neck Surgery
AAS	American Auditory Society
ACGIH	American Conference of Governmental Industrial Hygienists
ACOEM	American College of Occupational and Environmental Medicine
AGES	Age, Gene/Environment Susceptibility Study
AIHA	American Industrial Hygiene Association
ANSI	American National Standards Institute
ASHA	American Speech–Language–Hearing Association
BLS	Bureau of Labor Statistics
CAOHC	Council for Accreditation in Occupational Hearing Conservation
CDC	Centers for Disease Control and Prevention
CHABA	Committee on Hearing, Bioacoustics, and Biomechanics
CRADA	Cooperative Research and Development Agreement
DART	Division of Applied Research and Technology
DBBS	Division of Biomedical and Behavioral Sciences
DoD	Department of Defense

DPSE	Division of Physical Sciences and Engineering
DSHEFS	Division of Surveillance, Hazard Evaluations, and Field Studies
EID	Education and Information Division
EPA	Environmental Protection Agency
FTE	Full-time equivalent
FY	Fiscal year
HHE	Health Hazard Evaluation
HLPP	Hearing loss prevention program
HPD	Hearing protection device
INCE	Institute of Noise Control Engineering
IOM	Institute of Medicine
ISO	International Organization for Standardization
MSHA	Mine Safety and Health Administration
NASA	National Aeronautics and Space Administration
NHANES	National Health and Nutrition Examination Survey
NHCA	National Hearing Conservation Association
NIDCD	National Institute on Deafness and Other Communication Disorders
NIH	National Institutes of Health
NIHL	Noise-induced hearing loss
NIOSH	National Institute for Occupational Safety and Health
NORA	National Occupational Research Agenda
NRC	National Research Council
NRR	Noise Reduction Rating
NSF	National Science Foundation
NVLAP	National Voluntary Laboratory Accreditation Program
OEP	Office of Extramural Programs
OHC	Office of Health Communications
ORTT	Office of Research and Technology Transfer
OSHA	Occupational Safety and Health Administration
PA	Program Announcement
PRL	Pittsburgh Research Laboratory

r2p	Research to Practice
RFA	Request for Applications
SENSOR	Sentinel Event Notification System for Occupational Risks
SRL	Spokane Research Laboratory
STS	Standard threshold shift
UAW	United Automobile, Aerospace and Agricultural Implement Workers of America
USACHPPM	U.S. Army Center for Health Promotion and Preventive Medicine
WHO	World Health Organization

Summary

ABSTRACT *Occupational hearing loss is a serious concern for many workers, although the number affected is uncertain. Using data from the 1980s and 1990s, the National Institute for Occupational Safety and Health (NIOSH) estimated that at least 4 million workers in the United States were exposed to workplace noise levels that put them at risk of hearing loss. Some workers may also be at risk due to exposure to ototoxic chemicals. Occupational hearing loss may impede communication, contribute to safety hazards in the workplace, and adversely affect other aspects of workers' lives.*

In conjunction with planned reviews of up to 15 NIOSH research programs, the Institute of Medicine convened a committee of experts to review the NIOSH Hearing Loss Research Program to evaluate the relevance of its work to improvements in occupational safety and health and the impact of NIOSH research in reducing workplace illnesses and injuries. Relevance was evaluated in terms of the priority of work carried out and its connection to improvements in workplace protection. Impact was evaluated in terms of its contributions to worker health and safety. The committee was also asked to assess the program's identification and targeting of new research areas, to identify emerging research issues, and to provide advice on ways the program might be strengthened.

Although responsibility for controlling workplace exposures to noise or ototoxins lies with others, the Hearing Loss Research Program can be expected to contribute to efforts to reduce the effects of these workplace hazards through its research and information dissemination. Taking into account several important factors beyond the program's control, the committee found that over the past decade (the period covered by this review), the Hearing Loss Research Program has made meaningful contributions to improving worker health and safety.

Using a five-point scoring scale (where 5 is highest), the committee assigned the research program a score of 4 for impact, indicating that the program has made a moderate contribution on the basis of end outcomes (improvements in worker health or safety) or well-accepted intermediate outcomes (use or adoption of work by stakeholders). However, some of the program's work appears to be too narrowly targeted or directed to activities that are secondary to meeting the needs of protecting the hearing of workers. For this reason the committee assigned a score of 3 for relevance, indicating that often the research focuses on lesser priorities and is loosely or only indirectly connected to workplace protection.

To enhance the relevance and impact of its work and fulfill its stated mission of providing national and world leadership to reduce the prevalence of occupational hearing loss through a focused program of research and prevention, the committee recommends that the NIOSH Hearing Loss Research Program foster effective leadership in program planning and implementation; further implement program evaluation efforts; gain access to additional intramural and extramural expertise, especially in epidemiology and noise control engineering; and initiate and sustain efforts to obtain surveillance data for occupational hearing loss and workplace noise exposure.

The National Institute for Occupational Safety and Health (NIOSH) has included prevention of occupational hearing loss as part of its research portfolio since its establishment by the Occupational Safety and Health Act of 1970 (P.L. 91-596). Occupational hearing loss is a serious concern, although the number of workers affected is uncertain. Using data from the 1980s and early 1990s (the most recent available), NIOSH estimated that at least 4 million workers in the United States were exposed to workplace noise levels that put them at risk of hearing loss. Some workers may be at risk due to exposure to ototoxic chemicals. Occupational hearing loss may impede communication and contribute to safety hazards in the workplace, and it may adversely affect other aspects of workers' lives.

In conjunction with planned reviews of up to 15 NIOSH research programs, the Institute of Medicine (IOM) convened a committee of experts to review the NIOSH Hearing Loss Research Program to evaluate the relevance of its work to improvements in occupational safety and health and the impact of NIOSH research on reducing workplace illnesses and injuries. Relevance was evaluated in terms of the priority of work carried out and its connection to improvements in workplace protection. Research impact was evaluated in terms of its contributions to worker health and safety. The committee was also asked to assess the program's identification and targeting of new research areas, to identify emerging research issues, and to provide advice on ways the program might be strengthened.

As part of a research agency, the NIOSH Hearing Loss Research Program can engage in such activities as conducting and supporting research; developing surveillance programs; developing and disseminating recommendations and related tools to aid in implementing best practices to reduce hazardous noise exposure; and contributing to the education and training of employers, workers, and occupational health and safety professionals. Although the Hearing Loss Research Program has no authority to establish or enforce regulations on noise hazards and the prevention of occupational hearing loss, the program can be expected to contribute to efforts to reduce the effects of workplace hazards to hearing.

Overall, the committee found that over the past decade (the period covered by this review), the Hearing Loss Research Program has made meaningful contributions to improving worker health and safety. However, some of the program's work appears to be targeted too narrowly or directed to activities that are secondary to the goal of protecting the hearing of workers. To enhance the relevance and impact of the Hearing Loss Research Program's work and fulfill its stated mission of providing national and world leadership to reduce the prevalence of occupational hearing loss through a focused program of research and prevention, the committee urges several changes. The committee recommends that the NIOSH Hearing Loss Research Program take steps that include fostering effective leadership in program planning and implementation; further implementing program evaluation efforts; gaining access to additional intramural and extramural expertise, especially in epidemiology and noise control engineering; and initiating and sustaining efforts to obtain surveillance data for occupational hearing loss and workplace noise exposure.

STUDY PROCESS

The committee's review focused on the work of the NIOSH Hearing Loss Research Program primarily during the period 1996 through 2005.[1] The review

---

[1] The Hearing Loss Research Program is one of the first two research programs to be reviewed for NIOSH by National Academies committees. The review was conducted using evaluation guidance (referred to as the Framework Document) that was developed by the National Academies' Committee for Review of NIOSH Research Programs (the Framework Committee). The Framework Document appears in Appendix A.

was based largely on material that NIOSH Hearing Loss Research Program staff provided to the committee in oral presentations, a written evidence package, and written responses to questions from the committee.[2] The committee also received input from program stakeholders (see Chapter 1 and Appendix B), including representatives from labor, industry, regulatory agencies, professional organizations, and academia. The committee excluded nonauditory effects of noise from consideration.

As directed by its review guidance, the committee's evaluation included rating the relevance and impact of the Hearing Loss Research Program using five-point scales.

In evaluating relevance, the committee assessed the degree to which the program's research is in high-priority areas and is connected to improvements in workplace protection. To assign a summary rating, the committee decided to weight all of the program's activities nearly equally.

In evaluating impact, the committee assessed the degree to which the program's research can be shown to have made a contribution to improvements in worker health and safety. To assign a summary rating, the committee decided to consider the extent to which identifiable and worthwhile accomplishments could be shown, without discounting for lesser degrees of impact from some aspects of the program.

The committee's review was constrained by the lack of historical and current data on the nature and extent of occupational hearing loss or workplace noise exposures among U.S. workers. Data from surveillance programs or longitudinal studies of selected populations are needed to identify industrial sectors or workforce populations with the highest levels of occupational hearing loss or noise exposure and to identify improvements in these end outcomes.

FACTORS WITH BROAD EFFECTS ON THE HEARING LOSS RESEARCH PROGRAM

Several factors beyond the control of the Hearing Loss Research Program may have prevented it from working in an optimal way to achieve impact and relevance. Already noted is the need to rely on others to effect the changes in the workplace that are necessary to minimize hazardous noise environments and ensure worker compliance with hearing conservation programs. Other important factors are the program's matrix organization and small budget, congressional

---

[2]Some of the materials provided to the committee are available online at the NIOSH website *http://www.cdc.gov/niosh/nas/hlr/*.

earmarking of much of the program funding, and economic factors that employers may believe to be unfavorable to workplace implementation of noise control approaches to hearing loss prevention.

The Hearing Loss Research "Program" operates in a matrix environment, not as an identifiable entity in the NIOSH organization chart. The program comprises a collection of activities taking place principally within five organizationally separate and geographically distributed NIOSH units. Moreover, the Hearing Loss Research Program budget is small. In fiscal year (FY) 2005, the program had $5.2 million in intramural funding and $2.3 million in extramural funding, out of a total NIOSH budget of $286 million. Congressional direction as to the amount of the NIOSH budget to be applied to mining safety and health has significantly shaped the portfolio, staffing, and funding levels within the Hearing Loss Research Program. Funding that supports work related to noise control and prevention of hearing loss in the mining sector cannot be redirected to other Hearing Loss Research Program priorities. In FY 2005, this funding represented 69 percent of the Hearing Loss Research Program's total spending.

Over the course of its review, the committee also saw that the Hearing Loss Research Program is undergoing change as part of NIOSH's broader organizational changes and as a result of preparation for the IOM review. These changes have included identifying new research goals, naming new leadership, modifying the name of the program, and renaming one of its four research goals. Development of a strategic plan has been deferred until the conclusion of the IOM review.

HEARING LOSS RESEARCH PROGRAM MISSION AND GOALS

The stated mission of the Hearing Loss Research Program is to provide national and world leadership to reduce the prevalence of occupational hearing loss through a focused program of research and prevention.

In 2005, the Hearing Loss Research Program established four research goals:

1. Contribute to the Development, Implementation, and Evaluation of Effective Hearing Loss Prevention Programs
2. Reduce Hearing Loss Through Interventions Targeting Personal Protective Equipment
3. Develop Engineering Controls to Reduce Noise Exposures
4. Improve Understanding of Occupational Hearing Loss Through Surveillance and Investigation of Risk Factors

The Hearing Loss Research Program used these four goals to organize the primary evidence package provided to the committee. In turn, the committee used the four goals to organize its detailed examination of the program, while recognizing that these specific research goals were established only at the end of the period covered by the assessment.

ASSESSMENT OF RELEVANCE

Using the limited surveillance information available and members' expert judgment, the committee found that the Hearing Loss Research Program mission and four main research goals as stated were highly relevant to the overall aim of reducing occupational hearing loss. However, the committee identified several activities of lesser priority among the work carried out to pursue these goals, leading to considerable variation in relevance across the components of the program.

The program's efforts in development, implementation, and evaluation of effective hearing loss prevention programs (Research Goal 1) have addressed high-priority needs. The program has identified objectives and activities that, if pursued successfully, should prove to be highly relevant to the reduction of occupational hearing loss. However, increased emphasis is needed on evaluation of the components of hearing loss prevention programs, as well as on dissemination of materials to facilitate the development and application of engineering controls in prevention programs.

Research efforts on interventions targeting personal protective equipment (Research Goal 2) have focused primarily on two pressing problems: (1) more accurate representation in Noise Reduction Ratings of the workplace effectiveness of hearing protection devices and (2) evaluation of the fit and effectiveness of the devices during the work shift. The committee found this prioritization appropriate and adequately connected to improvements in workplace protection.

For engineering controls to reduce noise exposure (Research Goal 3), apportionment of effort within the discretionary budget of the Hearing Loss Program has not reflected their importance in the hierarchy of controls. Research efforts have been concentrated in the mining sector, with some attention to the construction sector. Miners are known to face serious noise hazards but represent a small proportion of the noise-exposed workforce. Although the committee considered the emphasis on mining, reflecting congressional direction, to be disproportionate to the distribution of workers exposed to noise hazards in other industrial sectors, this allocation is outside the control of the Hearing Loss Research Program. However, drawing on additional noise control engineering expertise, the program could and should take more aggressive steps both to apply and transfer technologies developed for the mining industry to other industry sectors and to develop noise control technology for other sectors.

The relevance of research efforts to improve understanding of occupational hearing loss through surveillance and investigation of risk factors (Research Goal 4) is mixed. The objective of establishing effective surveillance systems to monitor workers' noise exposures and incidence of hearing loss is highly relevant and requires increased attention, expertise, and priority from the Hearing Loss Research Program. However, the current and planned portfolio of surveillance activities is not focused on generating valid estimates of the number of individuals with occupational hearing loss, the risk of developing occupational hearing loss, or the distribution of noise exposure among workers. Investigation of the contribution of exposure to ototoxins to occupational hearing loss is appropriate, but the magnitude of the problem should be assessed. The committee judged efforts to elucidate the genetics of hearing loss and the role of the aging process unrelated to noise exposure as a diffusion of mission from worker safety. It would be more appropriate for these basic science questions to be pursued by other researchers outside of NIOSH. The program's expectations of benefit from audiometry data derived from surveys of the general population did not seem realistic.

The assessment of relevance also took into account the input and interests of stakeholders. Stakeholder involvement and input into NIOSH research prioritization were most apparent and laudable in the area of development, implementation, and evaluation of hearing loss prevention programs, at least as manifested in participation in conferences and workshops. With some exceptions noted elsewhere in this report, stakeholders (many of whom have partnered or collaborated with the Hearing Loss Research Program) submitted positive opinions to the committee about the relevance and appropriateness of the program's research efforts.

Overall, the committee found the activities of the Hearing Loss Research Program to include strong, high-priority work, as well as projects that the committee viewed to be of lesser priority. The committee was concerned that the program was not giving sufficient emphasis and priority to surveillance for occupational hearing loss and noise exposure, a fundamental gap in the field, or devoting enough breadth and expertise to its efforts in noise control engineering. In particular, the scope of Research Goal 3 was perceived as much too narrow, focused primarily on underground coal miners who constitute a small fraction of potentially noise-exposed industrial workers in the United States.

On the basis of its review, the committee assigned a score of 3 for the relevance of the NIOSH Hearing Loss Research Program. The five-point scale used for the rating of relevance is shown in Box S-1.

> **BOX S-1**
> **Scale for Rating Program Relevance**
>
> 5 = Research is in highest-priority subject areas and highly relevant to improvements in workplace protection; research results in, and NIOSH is engaged in, transfer activities at a significant level (highest rating).
> 4 = Research is in high-priority subject area and adequately connected to improvements in workplace protection; research results in, and NIOSH is engaged in, transfer activities.
> 3 = Research focuses on lesser priorities and is loosely or only indirectly connected to workplace protection; NIOSH is not significantly involved in transfer activities.
> 2 = Research program is not well integrated or well focused on priorities and is not clearly connected to workplace protection and inadequately connected to transfer activities.
> 1 = Research in the research program is an ad hoc collection of projects, is not integrated into a program, and is not likely to improve workplace safety or health.

ASSESSMENT OF IMPACT

End Outcomes

In trying to make judgments about the impact of work done by the Hearing Loss Research Program, the general lack of surveillance data on occupational hearing loss and noise exposures for U.S. workers during the past decade, as well as the lack of large, longitudinal intervention studies, meant that the committee was unable to consider evidence that the program has contributed to changes in end outcomes related to occupational hearing loss.

Intermediate Outcomes

Given the lack of data on changes in the end outcomes of occupational hearing loss and noise exposure, the committee based its assessment of the impact of the NIOSH Hearing Loss Research Program primarily on the evidence that its research products have been put to use beyond NIOSH in ways that have the potential to influence occupational hearing loss in the workplace. Evidence of these intermediate outcomes was available, in varying degrees, for all four research goals. In some instances, the committee also considered the potential for future impact from Hearing Loss Research Program publications and other program outputs that were not yet associated with intermediate outcomes.

Summary

The committee found that the Hearing Loss Research Program has made meaningful contributions through activities that include publication of intramural and extramural research findings in the peer-reviewed scientific literature, development of noise reduction methods and materials for the mining industry, collection and publication of resource materials for technical and lay audiences, development and delivery of educational programs, provision of technical advice to regulatory agencies, and participation of staff in the development of various national and international voluntary standards concerning noise and hearing loss.

The information provided by the Hearing Loss Research Program and comments from many stakeholders offer strong endorsement of the contributions made to efforts to reduce occupational hearing loss through work related to the development, implementation, and evaluation of effective hearing loss prevention programs (Research Goal 1). Many of the program's work products, including recommendations and training programs, have been adapted or adopted for use by business, labor, and occupational health professionals. However, the program has paid minimal attention to evaluating the effectiveness of these products in reducing the incidence or severity of occupational hearing loss or in achieving important intermediate outcomes such as sustained improvement in the use of hearing protection devices or the management of hearing loss prevention programs. Evaluation based on changes in knowledge, attitudes, or behavioral intentions is appropriate but not sufficient.

The committee found that the Hearing Loss Research Program has made important contributions to increasing knowledge about the real-world performance of hearing protection devices, improving the methods and tools for assessing hearing protector attenuation, and encouraging appropriate regulatory agencies and organizations to modify regulations and other guidance concerning hearing protector attenuation (Research Goal 2). The program's ability to help constituents in the field of hearing protection device regulation reach consensus around a standard method for measuring the real-ear attenuation of hearing protectors (ANSI [American National Standards Institute] S12.6–1997) has been especially noteworthy. Participation by Hearing Loss Research Program staff not only in intramural research but also in collaborations with other agencies and with academic scientists, hearing protector manufacturers, employers, and workers probably adds to the impact of the program in ways that are difficult to document.

The Hearing Loss Research Program is engaged in a narrow set of activities on engineering noise controls (Research Goal 3). These activities have had a limited impact and may have limited prospects for future impact. With a large share of this work taking place at the Pittsburgh Research Laboratory, the focus is primarily on engineering noise controls for mining. Mining equipment that incorporates the results of two projects pursued by Hearing Loss Research Program staff and their collaborators outside NIOSH is being produced and is in use in a small number of underground coal mines. The program has also contributed to efforts by the Mine Safety and Health Administration (MSHA) to identify technologically feasible and promising noise controls for use in mining.

The program's work on engineering noise controls appears to have had little impact in industrial sectors beyond mining. Development of the database on noise emission levels of powered hand tools can contribute information to users of these tools but makes no contribution to the development of engineering noise controls, either in the design of the products or in their use. In addition, the committee is concerned that the noise emission data were not generated using rigorous operational procedures in an accredited facility as would be expected for data collected for reference and decision-making purposes. Finally, although the development of noise control designs for power tools provided an opportunity for students at a few universities to gain experience in product noise control design, the value of this training experience probably does not outweigh the detractions of failing to aggressively pursue other approaches that are needed to promote the development of robust and effective solutions that could attract industry participation and implementation in the marketplace.

The work being done to improve understanding of occupational hearing loss through surveillance and investigation of risk factors (Research Goal 4) has been directed in large part to data gathering, epidemiologic studies, and studies using laboratory animals to investigate the causative mechanisms of hearing loss. Over the past decade an increasing proportion of the work has been done by extramural researchers. The impact of this research occurs primarily through its contributions to the knowledge base on occupational hearing loss. The program's work on ototoxicity is widely cited by other researchers and is reflected in the hearing conservation policies of some organizations. The program's support for the Occupational Safety and Health Administration's (OSHA's) implementation in 2004 of separate reporting of recordable occupational hearing loss has contributed to generating at least a minimal form of surveillance data. Other work conducted in conjunction with this program area is likely to make some contribution to basic knowledge regarding genetic and age-related aspects of hearing loss but will not readily contribute to knowledge regarding noise exposure and hearing loss among workers. For this as well as other research areas, the limited number of peer-reviewed publications and a lack of timeliness in publishing key research findings and important workshop proceedings were of concern to the committee.

On the basis of its review, the committee assigned the NIOSH Hearing Loss Research Program a score of 4 for impact, notwithstanding significant shortcomings in some aspects of the program. The five-point scale used for the rating of impact is shown in Box S-2.

> **BOX S-2**
> **Scale for Rating Program Impact**
>
> 5 = Research program has made a major contribution to worker health and safety on the basis of end outcomes or well-accepted intermediate outcomes.
> 4 = Research program has made a moderate contribution on the basis of end outcomes or well-accepted intermediate outcomes; research program generated important new knowledge and is engaged in transfer activities, but well-accepted intermediate outcomes or end outcomes have not been documented.
> 3 = Research program activities or outputs are going on and are likely to produce improvements in worker health and safety (with explanation of why not rated higher).
> 2 = Research program activities or outputs are going on and may result in new knowledge or technology, but only limited application is expected.
> 1 = Research activities and outputs are NOT likely to have any application.
> NA = Impact cannot be assessed; program is not mature enough.

IDENTIFYING EMERGING ISSUES AND RESEARCH AREAS

In addition to evaluating the relevance and impact of the work of the NIOSH Hearing Loss Research Program to health and safety in the workplace, the committee is charged with assessing the program's targeting of new research areas and identification of emerging issues in occupational safety and health most relevant to future improvements in workplace protection.

The Hearing Loss Research Program's Identification of Emerging Issues and Research Areas in Occupational Hearing Loss

The NIOSH Hearing Loss Research Program identified 12 emerging research issues distributed across its four current research goals. Two activities figured prominently in the program's recent efforts to identify research needs: a Futures Workshop in April 2005 and the development of the Mining Health and Safety Research Program Plan. The Futures Workshop was planned as a way to develop research goals for the Hearing Loss Research Program for the next 5 to 10 years.

Acknowledging the small scale of the Hearing Loss Research Program and other challenges noted earlier, the committee nonetheless has concerns about the program's identification of new or emerging research. With few exceptions, the emerging issues resemble the work that the program described elsewhere as being under way or among its current research goals. In the committee's view, the limited nature of the emerging issues identified by the Hearing Loss Research Program may reflect two problems. One is limited outreach to and input from communities responsible for preventing occupational hearing loss regarding the development of a research agenda. The other problem is the challenge of setting research priorities while having only minimal data on the occurrence of work-related hearing loss and workers' exposure to noise and/or ototoxic chemicals.

The committee sees a need for much wider outreach for input and ideas to guide the direction of future work by the Hearing Loss Research Program. Areas of expertise where the committee particularly urges seeking greater outside contact include engineering noise control, low-noise product design, epidemiology, and program evaluation.

Similarly, targeting research efforts without having adequate current information about the epidemiology of work-related hearing loss is necessarily limiting. Although establishing surveillance programs for occupational hearing loss and noise exposure and conducting a large epidemiologic survey of industry are listed as long-term research topics, these activities need to be given higher priority because of the fundamental role of the data they will generate in the research planning process.

Emerging Research Needs Identified by the Evaluation Committee

The committee was asked to identify emerging research needs in occupational hearing loss and noise control. Given the short time frame for this review, the committee identified a limited number of topics and reviewed suggestions from stakeholders (see Chapter 3), but it could not undertake a comprehensive assessment of the field.

RECOMMENDATIONS FOR PROGRAM IMPROVEMENT

As the only federal research program focused specifically on the challenge of preventing occupational hearing loss, the NIOSH Hearing Loss Research Program should be an undisputed leader and source of expertise in the fields of occupational hearing loss research, including hearing loss prevention programs, hearing protection, noise control engineering for occupational hearing loss prevention, and occupational hearing loss surveillance and risk factors. The committee identified several potential opportunities to improve the relevance of the program's work and strengthen its impact on reducing occupational hearing loss. A summary of the committee's recommendations appears in Box S-3.

The committee recognizes that some of these recommendations carry resource implications that have not been fully explored. It hopes that NIOSH will place a high enough value on the Hearing Loss Research Program to give serious consideration to finding ways to respond to these opportunities for improvement.

Program Management in a Matrix Environment

The NIOSH Hearing Loss Research Program operates in a matrix environment, which poses challenges for the program's ability to develop and implement a program plan and to allocate resources in accordance with program priorities. Even the most talented leadership will find it difficult to successfully manage a program distributed across separate organizational units and to catalyze the planning and mobilization of resources necessary for a cohesive program. The small size of the program also demands skill in setting priorities for program activities and use of program resources. The program as a whole and each of the four research program areas require leadership specifically dedicated to championing a better Hearing Loss Research Program. In addition to having excellent management skills, leaders should be well-regarded experts in hearing loss prevention, noise control engineering, or surveillance methods, with experience in implementing hearing loss prevention or noise control engineering practices in the field.

Since 1996, the Hearing Loss Research Program has had to respond to significant organizational and leadership challenges. Although the program has persevered admirably during these transitional times, the committee sees a need to foster leadership that can provide coherence to the program, increase collaboration, and serve as an effective advocate within the matrix environment in which it operates. The committee is encouraged to see that NIOSH has recently appointed from within the NIOSH management staff an overall program manager who is expected to monitor the program's activities and resources. In this role, the program manager will have an advisory and consultative relationship with the organizational units in which the Hearing Loss Research Program's work is done, but he will not have authority to mandate the allocation of resources to the program as a whole or its components. The program manager did not make a formal presentation to the committee, and even though he is new to this position, it would have been valuable to the committee to hear his views on the program and the IOM review.

1. **Foster effective leadership.** NIOSH should ensure that the Hearing Loss Research Program and its components have leadership with appropriate technical expertise as well as skills in managing in a complex environment, mobilizing resources, promoting collaboration within the program, and increasing program coherence. All of these leaders must serve as champions of the program within and outside NIOSH

and help to garner adequate resources and recruit expertise. The leaders should be respected and involved in the hearing loss prevention community and in their own fields of expertise. NIOSH should provide the overall program leader with sufficient authority to make appropriate program and budgetary decisions.

The leaders of the Hearing Loss Research Program must contend with a small budget—about $7.5 million in FY 2005—much of which is reserved for work related to mining or for extramural research. The committee urges NIOSH to consider the need for program resources that are commensurate with a more robust pursuit of the program's goals and with sustaining the continuity of the most relevant research in specific program areas.

Access to Intramural and Extramural Expertise

The committee is concerned that the Hearing Loss Research Program has lacked adequate internal technical expertise, especially in the specialized areas of epidemiology and noise control engineering, and has appeared to rely on a fairly narrow group of external experts for input and collaboration. For the program to hold the position of national leadership, it must draw upon outstanding members of the communities responsible for the prevention of occupational hearing loss both within and outside the program.

As the Hearing Loss Research Program garners additional internal expertise, it should also broaden and strengthen its ties to sources of external scientific, hearing loss prevention, and noise control engineering expertise, such as other federal agencies, industry, and the military. With additional expertise, the program will be better positioned to have an impact on occupational hearing loss through its current portfolio as well as to move into emerging research areas for the future.

2. **Recruit additional expert researchers to the NIOSH Hearing Loss Research Program staff.** The Hearing Loss Research Program should recruit and retain experienced professionals with recognized expertise in the fields of epidemiology and noise control engineering who can exercise leadership in planning, conducting, and evaluating the program's work in these crucial areas. It is essential for the program to make gaining this additional expertise a priority.
3. **Expand access to outside expertise.** The program should make efforts to draw more broadly from the communities responsible for the prevention of occupational hearing loss as reviewers, conference participants, and collaborators. As part of this effort, the program should

strengthen ties to the National Institute on Deafness and Other Communication Disorders and other components of the National Institutes of Health to benefit from additional interactions with the scientific researchers there. The program should also explore expanding its collaborations with noise control engineers inside and outside the federal government.

Program Planning

Even as the National Academies' evaluation of up to 15 different NIOSH research programs is under way, NIOSH as a whole is undergoing changes. NIOSH has reorganized its research portfolio into sector and cross-sector programs and coordinated emphasis areas. It is developing strategic plans for each of its research programs, and new emphasis is being placed on the translation and application of scientific knowledge to the workplace. The committee commends NIOSH for its continued striving for improvement as an organization.

The Hearing Loss Research Program has acknowledged that until recently it has managed more by opportunity than by objective. Although it may not be feasible for such a small program to manage entirely by objective, and the group has proven itself adept at leveraging opportunities, the committee urges additional efforts to focus its limited resources on specific goals, with input from surveillance data, evaluation of the effectiveness of its program activities, regulatory agencies, and other stakeholders.

4. **Develop a strategic plan.** The Hearing Loss Research Program should develop a strategic plan that takes into account the strengths, weaknesses, and external factors identified in this evaluation. It should reflect a focus on the program's mission and serve to guide decision making about the value of projects and proposed collaborations. It should also reflect coordination with the strategic plans developed by the sector-based NIOSH research programs that may need to address hearing loss as one of several health hazards faced by the workforce.
5. **Use surveillance data as well as stakeholder input to identify priorities.** The Hearing Loss Research Program should make the rationale for its research prioritization more explicit, using analyses of surveillance data to the extent possible as well as the concerns and interests of stakeholders from a variety of industrial sectors to guide allocations of resources and effort.
6. **Use information from evaluation of hearing loss prevention measures to guide program planning.** The Hearing Loss Research Pro-

gram should use information gained from evaluation of the effectiveness of its program activities to help identify approaches to hearing loss prevention that should be emphasized, revised, or possibly discontinued.

7. **Systematize collaboration with regulatory partners.** The Hearing Loss Research Program should establish regular means for conferring with OSHA, MSHA, and the Environmental Protection Agency to better anticipate research needs relevant to regulatory decision making.

Evaluation of Hearing Loss Prevention Measures

Developing and disseminating "best practices" and training methods for hearing loss prevention programs to apply scientific understanding to the workplace has been an important contribution of the Hearing Loss Research Program and is the focus of Research Goal 1. The program noted the need for intervention effectiveness research designed to validate best practices for each of the seven components of hearing loss prevention programs it advocates. The committee underscores the importance of evaluation of the effectiveness of all program activities, including the dissemination of the educational material that the program develops, as a crucial step in ensuring that the Hearing Loss Research Program serves as a leader in producing evidence-based guidance on hearing loss prevention.

8. **Place greater emphasis on evaluation of the effectiveness of hearing loss prevention measures on the basis of outcomes that are as closely related as possible to reducing noise exposure and the incidence of occupational hearing loss.** The Hearing Loss Research Program should implement consistent and concerted evaluation activities that inform and focus its work on hearing loss prevention. Prospective evaluations of the recommended components of hearing loss prevention programs are needed to determine which features have the most significant impacts on reducing noise exposure levels or hearing loss incidence rates. These evaluations should address actual (not just intended) worker and employer behavior and the end results of exposure levels and hearing loss.

Surveillance Activities

The Hearing Loss Research Program identified the lack of surveillance data for workers' noise exposures and the incidence and severity of occupational hearing loss as one of the fundamental knowledge gaps in the field. The committee agrees and underscores the importance of surveillance data and their careful analysis to help guide priority setting for research in occupational health and safety and for evaluation of program activities. Although the Hearing Loss Research Program has participated in several different efforts to address the lack of surveillance data, the program's current approaches are piecemeal and require expansion of their conceptual framework and measurement methods. To maintain an appropriate scientific leadership role in the field of occupational hearing loss prevention, the Hearing Loss Research Program needs to increase its emphasis on and expertise in surveillance. Doing so will require resources commensurate with the task, as well as the leadership of one or more experienced epidemiologists integrated into the program staff. Relying on ad hoc epidemiologic assistance is not sufficient. With that additional expertise, the Hearing Loss Research Program should plan means to gather and analyze new data on the occurrence of hearing loss and hazardous noise exposure.

9. **Initiate national surveillance for occupational hearing loss and hazardous noise.** The Hearing Loss Research Program should rally expertise and resources to lead surveillance of the incidence and prevalence of work-related hearing loss and the occurrence of exposure to hazardous noise levels in occupational settings in the United States. Surveillance efforts should be accompanied by plans for appropriate analyses of the data.

Noise Control Perspective

Following the industrial hygiene tradition of the "hierarchy of controls," noise control engineering should be the primary approach to prevention of hearing loss. In reality, employers frequently turn first to administrative controls or hearing protection devices to decrease workers' exposure to hazardous noise. Perhaps as a result, the research emphasis within the Hearing Loss Research Program has also been on aspects of hearing loss prevention other than noise control. Over the past decade, substantially more of the program's resources have been brought to bear on noise control engineering, but those resources have been directed primarily to the mining industry. Although congressional guidance has resulted in most of this funding being devoted to a single industrial sector, the committee sees it as the mission of the Hearing Loss Research Program to pursue broader applications of its work on noise control engineering. To help identify the potential for broader applications of mining-related work, the committee urges increased collaboration between the Pittsburgh- and Cincinnati-based researchers.

10. **Integrate the noise control engineering perspective into overall program efforts for all sectors.** The Hearing Loss Research Program should apply its dissemination expertise to further emphasize the application of "quiet by design," "buy quiet," and engineered noise control approaches to industrial settings as part of hearing loss prevention programs.
11. **Develop noise control engineering approaches for non-mining sectors.** The Hearing Loss Research Program should increase efforts to develop noise control approaches applicable in industrial sectors outside mining where workers are also at risk from hazardous noise. Where possible, "dual-use" applications from work done in mining could help bring noise reduction benefit to both miners and workers from other industrial sectors.
12. **Increase the visibility of noise control engineering as a component of the Hearing Loss Research Program.** The Hearing Loss Research Program should use means such as periodic workshops on noise control engineering topics to raise the visibility of its noise control engineering projects within the field. Such workshops can facilitate information exchange, can provide specialized technical training, and may attract qualified professionals who can serve as advisers, consultants, collaborators, or recruits to the NIOSH program.
13. **Accredit laboratories used to conduct studies for the Hearing Loss Research Program.** The Hearing Loss Research Program should work to achieve accreditation of all laboratories that are involved in the acquisition of data that are published or shared externally. To the extent possible, testing on behalf of the NIOSH intramural program should be carried out at facilities owned or controlled by NIOSH.

Extramural Research

Between FY 1997 and FY 2005, slightly more than $14 million, about 30 percent of the total expenditures of the NIOSH Hearing Loss Program, was directed toward extramural projects related to hearing loss or noise control engineering. With the exception of one Request for Application (RFA) in 2001, the program has relied on investigator-initiated proposals. The extramural research that has resulted includes important contributions to the knowledge base in this field and has facilitated some productive collaborations with Hearing Loss Research Program researchers. In some cases, however, intramural researchers have not made themselves aware of relevant extramural research, which may have resulted in limited opportunities for effective collaboration.

In addition, greater use of RFAs and focused Program Announcements (PAs) has the potential to direct some extramural funding toward high-priority research topics that complement the intramural work. The Hearing Loss Research Program may also want to further pursue efforts to invite outside researchers to work at NIOSH facilities on a temporary basis and at little cost to the program. The committee recommends the following steps to maximize the benefit that extramural funding might bring to realizing the mission of the Hearing Loss Research Program:

14. **Target more of the extramural research funding.** The Hearing Loss Research Program should increase its use of Requests for Applications and focused Program Announcements to target more of its extramural research funding toward program priority areas.
15. **Increase collaboration and mutual awareness of ongoing work among intramural and extramural researchers.** For the Hearing Loss Research Program to maximize the benefit of extramural research, it is important for intramural and extramural researchers to each be aware of the work that the others are doing relevant to occupational hearing loss or noise control. Where appropriate, intramural researchers should be building upon extramural work within the Hearing Loss Research Program. Toward this end, after a grant has been awarded, NIOSH should facilitate increased communication between intra- and extramural researchers.

BOX S-3
Summary of Recommendations

Program Management in a Matrix Environment

Foster effective leadership.

Access to Intramural and Extramural Expertise

Recruit additional expert researchers to the NIOSH Hearing Loss Research Program staff.
Expand access to outside expertise.

Program Planning

Develop a strategic plan.
Use surveillance data as well as stakeholder input to identify priorities.
Use information from evaluation of hearing loss prevention measures to guide program planning.
Systematize collaboration with regulatory partners.

Evaluation of Hearing Loss Prevention Measures

Place greater emphasis on evaluation of the effectiveness of hearing loss prevention measures on the basis of outcomes that are as closely related as possible to reducing noise exposure and the incidence of occupational hearing loss.

Surveillance Activities

Initiate national surveillance for occupational hearing loss and hazardous noise.

Noise Control Perspective

Integrate the noise control engineering perspective into overall program efforts for all sectors.
Develop noise control engineering approaches for non-mining sectors.
Increase the visibility of noise control engineering as a component of the Hearing Loss Research Program.
Accredit laboratories used to conduct studies for the Hearing Loss Research Program.

Extramural Research

Target more of the extramural research funding.
Increase collaboration and mutual awareness of ongoing work among intramural and extramural researchers.

1

Introduction

The National Institute for Occupational Safety and Health (NIOSH) was established by the Occupational Safety and Health Act of 1970 (U.S. Congress, 1970). Today the agency is part of the Centers for Disease Control and Prevention of the U.S. Department of Health and Human Services. NIOSH is charged with the responsibility to "conduct . . . research, experiments, and demonstrations relating to occupational safety and health" and to develop "innovative methods, techniques, and approaches for dealing with [those] problems" (U.S. Congress, 1970). Its research targets include identifying criteria for use in setting worker exposure standards and exploring new problems that may arise in the workplace. NIOSH does not have the authority to establish or enforce regulations on workplace safety and health. Regulatory and enforcement authority rests with such agencies as the Occupational Safety and Health Administration (OSHA) and the Mine Safety and Health Administration (MSHA).

Prevention of occupational hearing loss has been part of the NIOSH research portfolio from the time the agency was established. A principal cause of occupational hearing loss is the cumulative effect of years of exposure to hazardous noise.[1]

---

[1] NIOSH considers workplace exposure to 8-hour time-weighted average noise levels of 85 dBA or higher or any exposure to levels of 140 dB SPL (sound pressure level) or higher to be hazardous to hearing (NIOSH, 1998).

Exposure to certain chemicals with or without concomitant noise exposure may also contribute to occupational hearing loss. Hearing loss may impede communication in the workplace and contribute to safety hazards. Occupationally acquired hearing loss may also have an adverse effect on workers' lives beyond the workplace. No medical means are currently available to prevent or reverse it, although hearing aids are widely used and research on other treatments is ongoing.

Occupational hearing loss is a serious concern, although the number of workers affected is uncertain. Determining the magnitude of the problem has been a persistent challenge because of the lack of national surveillance systems or more narrowly focused longitudinal studies to track workplace exposures to noise or ototoxic chemicals and the incidence or severity of hearing loss among workers. Under new OSHA requirements, implemented in 2004, employers are expected for the first time to record qualifying cases of occupational hearing loss separately from any other illness or injury. This reporting change will help generate welcome data on occupational hearing loss, but those data still have important limitations (see Chapter 2).

Using data from the 1980s and early 1990s, NIOSH estimated that at least 4 million workers in the United States were exposed to workplace noise levels that put them at risk of hearing loss (NIOSH, 1998). Other unpublished analyses suggested that the number may have been as high as 30 million in the early 1990s (NIOSH, 1996). Some workers may also be at risk due to exposure to ototoxic chemicals (NIOSH, 1996, 2005a). In addition, workers may be exposed to hearing hazards through noisy recreational activities (e.g., hunting, woodworking) and may develop hearing loss due to injury, illness, and aging.

A variety of disciplines or areas of expertise are involved in the prevention of occupational hearing loss. Practitioners in industrial hygiene, audiology (specifically occupational audiology), occupational medicine and nursing, noise control engineering, and safety engineering all play roles, as do epidemiologists and basic science researchers studying noise exposure and hearing loss. In addition, certain businesses share an interest in developing technologies for hearing loss prevention. Throughout this report, these groups are described as the communities responsible for occupational hearing loss prevention.

STUDY CHARGE AND EVALUATION COMMITTEE

In September 2004, NIOSH requested that the National Academies conduct reviews of as many as 15 NIOSH programs with respect to the impact and relevance of their work in reducing workplace injury and illness and to identify future directions that their work might take. The Hearing Loss Research Program was selected by NIOSH as one of the first two programs to be reviewed.

INTRODUCTION

The Committee to Review the NIOSH Hearing Loss Research Program was convened by the Institute of Medicine (IOM) in late 2005. The Statement of Task for the committee is as follows:

> The National Institute for Occupational Safety and Health (NIOSH) has requested that the National Research Council (NRC) and the Institute of Medicine review as many as 15 of its programs with respect to their impact, relevance, and future directions. Each program review will be conducted by a separate committee. The IOM will convene the Committee to Review the NIOSH Hearing Loss Research Program.
>
> The committee will examine the following issues for the Hearing Loss Research Program:
>
> (1) Progress in reducing workplace illness and injuries through occupational safety and health research, assessed on the basis of an analysis of relevant data about workplace illnesses and injuries and an evaluation of the effect that NIOSH research has had in reducing illness and injuries.
>
> (2) Progress in targeting new research to the areas of occupational safety and health most relevant to future improvements in workplace protection.
>
> (3) Significant emerging research areas that appear especially important in terms of their relevance to the mission of NIOSH.
>
> The committee will evaluate the Hearing Loss Research Program using an assessment framework developed by the NRC/IOM Committee to Review the NIOSH Research Programs. The evaluation will consider what the NIOSH program is producing as well as whether the program can reasonably be credited with changes in workplace practices, or whether such changes are the result of other factors unrelated to NIOSH. For cases where impact is difficult to measure directly, the committee reviewing the Hearing Loss Research Program may use information on intermediate outcomes to evaluate performance.

The study committee was selected to include members with expertise in audiology, biological mechanisms of noise-induced hearing loss and ototoxicity, noise control engineering, occupational health and safety, hearing conservation programs, epidemiology, and program evaluation. Committee members have varied experience in settings such as academia, industry, labor unions, and federal and state agencies charged with monitoring and regulating worker health and safety.

As specified in the Statement of Task, the committee performed its review using evaluation guidance, referred to as the Framework Document, which was developed by the National Academies' Committee for Review of NIOSH Research Programs. (The Framework Document is included as Appendix A of this report.) The study committee was given the discretion to determine the period to be covered by the review and chose to focus on the period since 1996 because it coincided with important organizational changes in the Hearing Loss Research Program and the introduction of the National Occupational Research Agenda (NORA). In relation to noise hazards, the review task was interpreted as applying only to hearing loss because of the name and mission of the program under review. Consideration of possible nonauditory health effects of noise exposure was excluded.

The committee met three times from January 2006 through March 2006 and conducted additional deliberations through four conference calls and e-mail. In addition, a subset of the committee visited facilities used by the NIOSH Hearing Loss Research Program staff at the Pittsburgh Research Laboratory and the Robert A. Taft Laboratory in Cincinnati, Ohio. Committee members also visited facilities at the University of Cincinnati, where testing of powered hand tool noise emissions is being done under contract to NIOSH.

The committee's review of the NIOSH Hearing Loss Research Program was based in large part on written materials provided by NIOSH (see Appendix C).[2] Information gathering included presentations made by NIOSH staff and other invited guests in open sessions of committee meetings in January and February (see Appendix B). The committee also invited comments from stakeholders, that is, organizations and individuals with a potential interest in the NIOSH Hearing Loss Research Program. The population of potential stakeholders is diverse and not easily defined. As a result, the committee made an effort to reach a varied national and international audience in federal and state agencies, industry, labor, and academia, but could not attempt to make this information-gathering effort a comprehensive or systematic survey of the program's stakeholders because of the short time frame for its work. (Additional detail on committee methods and a list of stakeholders who provided information to the committee are available in Appendix B.)

THE NIOSH HEARING LOSS RESEARCH PROGRAM

The NIOSH Hearing Loss Research Program describes its mission as "to provide national and world leadership to reduce the prevalence of occupational hear-

---

[2]Some of the materials provided to the committee are available online at the NIOSH website *http://www.cdc.gov/niosh/nas/hlr/*.

ing loss through a focused program of research and prevention" (NIOSH, 2005a). The following overview of the program is based on information provided to the committee by NIOSH.

History of the NIOSH Hearing Loss Research Program

One of the earliest products of the Hearing Loss Research Program was the publication in 1972 of *Criteria for a Recommended Standard: Occupational Exposure to Noise* (NIOSH, 1972), which provided the basis for a recommended standard to reduce the risk of developing permanent hearing loss as a result of occupational noise exposure. This work made an important contribution to the noise exposure standard for general industry promulgated by OSHA in the early 1980s. NIOSH published its first compendium of hearing protection devices in 1976, and in 1990 first published *Preventing Occupational Hearing Loss: A Practical Guide*.

The Hearing Loss Research Program was originally based in Cincinnati, Ohio. The program staff was part of the Physical Agents Effects Branch in the Division of Biomedical and Behavioral Sciences (DBBS). In 2000, DBBS and the Division of Physical Sciences and Engineering (DPSE) were merged to form the Division of Applied Research and Technology (DART). After the merger, most of the Cincinnati-based intramural activities were conducted by personnel in the Engineering and Physical Hazards Branch of DART. The Engineering and Physical Hazards Branch resulted from the merger of what had been the DBBS Physical Agents Effects Branch and the DPSE Engineering Control Technology Branch. The researchers and laboratories did not change location (NIOSH, 2006c).

In 1996, personnel and facilities, including research laboratories in Pittsburgh and Spokane, were transferred to NIOSH from the disestablished U.S. Bureau of Mines (NIOSH, 2005a). At the time, the Bureau of Mines had a small research effort on hearing loss prevention in the mining sector. The NIOSH Hearing Loss Research Program expanded to include activities based at the Pittsburgh Research Laboratory (PRL) and to a limited extent at the Spokane Research Laboratory (SRL). Initially, only about three researchers were involved in hearing loss research at PRL (Lotz, 2006a; NIOSH, 2006d). With growth of the research team in Pittsburgh, a Hearing Loss Prevention Branch was established at PRL in 2003.

Hearing Loss Research Program Structure

As of 2006, four NIOSH divisions and three NIOSH offices are involved in the Hearing Loss Research Program (NIOSH, 2005a):

- Division of Applied Research and Technology (DART)
- Pittsburgh Research Laboratory (PRL)
- Division of Surveillance, Hazard Evaluations, and Field Studies (DSHEFS)
- Education and Information Division (EID)
- Office of Extramural Programs (OEP)
- Office of Health Communications (OHC)
- Office of Research and Technology Transfer (ORTT)

The current organizational configuration of NIOSH is shown in Figure 1-1, and units specifically engaged in activities that are part of the Hearing Loss Research Program are highlighted in Figure 1-2. This distribution of activities across organizational units means that the program functions as a matrix organization, in which the people who carry out the work of the program are assigned to divisions and laboratories throughout the organization, rather than operating as an administrative entity within NIOSH.

Goals, Objectives, and Future Plans as Presented by NIOSH

As noted above, the mission of the Hearing Loss Research Program is to provide national and world leadership to reduce the prevalence of occupational hearing loss through a focused program of research and prevention (NIOSH, 2005a).

A revised noise criteria document prepared by the program and published in 1998 (NIOSH, 1998) identified the following research needs in occupational hearing loss:

- Noise Control
- Impulsive Noise
- Nonauditory Effects of Noise
- Auditory Effects of Ototoxic Chemical Exposures
- Exposure Monitoring
- Hearing Protectors
- Training and Motivation
- Program Evaluation
- Rehabilitation

Between 1998, when these goals were articulated, and 2005, the Hearing Loss Research Program sought to advance research in each area except the nonauditory effects of noise. Program staff reported to the committee that this area was not addressed because of the conflicting data in the published literature and the staff's

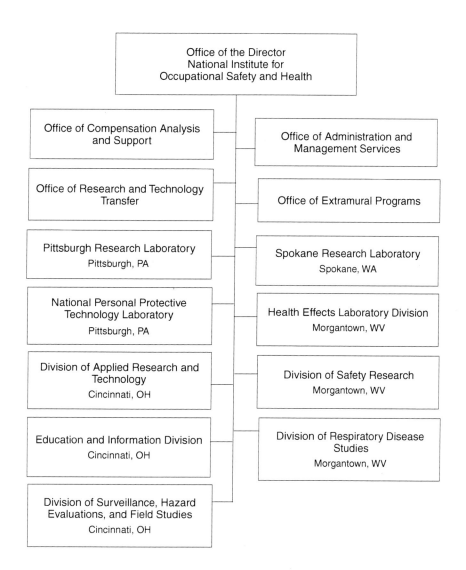

FIGURE 1-1 NIOSH organization chart, as of December 2005. SOURCE: NIOSH, 2005b.

need to prioritize the allocation of limited resources. NIOSH also considered that research activities directed at reducing noise exposure and its auditory effects would help prevent any nonauditory effects of exposure.

During this period, the Hearing Loss Research Program was also influenced by the broader NIOSH agenda. In 1996, using input received from the occupational health and safety community at large, NIOSH developed NORA. Under NORA, 21

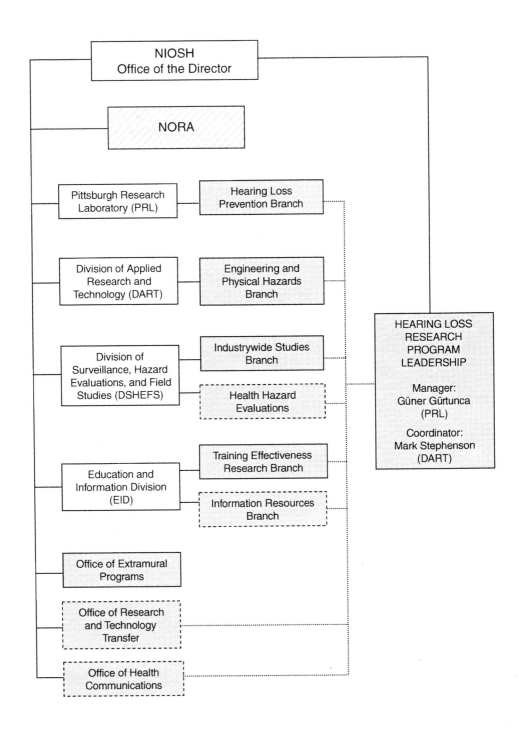

topics were identified as priority areas, with "hearing loss" and "mixed exposures" being the two areas in which the Hearing Loss Research Program was primarily involved. The program has also done work related to the NORA priority topics "control technology and personal protective equipment," "exposure assessment methods," and "intervention effectiveness research" (NIOSH, 2005a).

In 2000, the Hearing Loss Research Program, informed by input from NORA participants, successfully developed a proposal for NORA funding for a coordinated set of projects for fiscal years (FY) 2001–2005. The proposal was designed to address gaps in the overall research program and emphasized the mining and construction sectors (NIOSH, 2005a).

The work on hearing loss prevention done at PRL also falls under the purview of the NIOSH Mining Safety and Health Research Program. In the past few years, this program developed a strategic plan—the Mining Research Plan—that includes the following as one of its goals: "Reduce noise-induced hearing loss (NIHL) in the mining industry." Intermediate goals and corresponding performance measures were defined for this and other strategic goals in the plan (see Chapter 3) (NIOSH, 2005a).

In 2004, the Hearing Loss Research Program began its own strategic planning effort to coincide with the end of its 5-year NORA activities and the announcement of a new alignment of NIOSH research programs. A Futures Workshop was held in April 2005 "to bring stakeholders and internal and external researchers

FIGURE 1-2 Location of Hearing Loss Research Program activities in NIOSH. The Hearing Loss Research Program operates as a matrix organization, with its activities conducted in several NIOSH units. Units involved in carrying out activities of the Hearing Loss Research Program are shaded. The units conducting or providing funding for program activities are shown with solid borders. Units supporting program activities other than research are indicated by dashed borders. The program is overseen by a manager and coordinator who are based within administrative units, as indicated in the figure. Other units are shown to indicate the administrative relationship between the units involved in the Hearing Loss Research Program and the NIOSH organizational structure. NORA is not an administrative unit as such, but it is a program that is a potential source of funding and priorities for the Hearing Loss Research Program. Solid lines connect units with formal administrative relationships, and dotted lines represent advisory or consultative relationships. The Hearing Loss Research Program leadership is designated by and responsible to the NIOSH director, and it acts through advisory and consultative relationships with various NIOSH units. NOTE: NORA, National Occupational Research Agenda. SOURCE: NIOSH, 2005a; Lotz, 2006b,c.

together to discuss emerging topics and priorities" (NIOSH, 2005a). The program's strategic planning effort has been deferred until the conclusion of this IOM evaluation. The Futures Workshop and identification of emerging research needs are discussed further in Chapter 3.

One outgrowth of the Futures Workshop, however, was the adoption in 2005 of four new research goals to describe the current scope of the Hearing Loss Research Program's activities:

1. Contribute to the Development, Implementation, and Evaluation of Effective Hearing Loss Prevention Programs
2. Reduce Hearing Loss Through Interventions Targeting Personal Protective Equipment
3. Develop Engineering Controls to Reduce Noise Exposures
4. Contribute to Reductions in Hearing Loss Through the Understanding of Causative Mechanisms

The research topics that the program had pursued since 1998 are encompassed under these new goals. NIOSH used the four goals to organize the material provided to the committee, and the committee in turn used them to conduct its review (see Chapter 2). In early 2006, the Hearing Loss Research Program changed Goal 4 to "Improve Understanding of Occupational Hearing Loss Through Surveillance and Investigation of Risk Factors."

In 2006, NIOSH launched the second decade of NORA, replacing the 21 priority research areas established in 1996 with a sector-based approach to its research portfolio and to developing partnerships and obtaining input from stakeholders. NIOSH and its partners will form Research Councils for eight industry sectors: agriculture, forestry, and fishing; mining; construction; manufacturing; wholesale and retail trade; transportation, warehousing, and utilities; services; and health care and social assistance. "Hearing loss prevention" is one of 15 cross-sector programs under the new organization.

Program Resources

Staffing

Approximately 40 full-time equivalent positions, including contributions from 30 professional staff members, are currently involved in the intramural hearing loss research effort. This team includes 14 engineers, 5 audiologists, 4 psychologists, and single representatives of other professional disciplines, including physics, industrial hygiene, geology, nursing, sociology, computer science, and scientific communication. The staff is distributed among research teams in Cincinnati and Pittsburgh, with roughly half of the research staff and the program manager located in Pittsburgh.

Funding

Displayed in Table 1-1 is annual funding for intramural and extramural activities under the Hearing Loss Research Program for the period 1997–2005.

Intramural funding supports staff salaries and benefits, as well as contracts for goods and services related to staff research activities. The Hearing Loss Research Program also receives support for intramural work through interagency collaborations and participates in cooperative research and development agreements (CRADAs) with private companies to work cooperatively in technology development efforts.

As a result of the matrix nature of the Hearing Loss Research Program, the program's intramural funding level is the sum of the financial resources that the individual NIOSH organizational units decide to apply to work on hearing loss prevention or noise control activities. During the period covered by this review, the largest portion of the program's intramural funding—69 percent in FY 2005—has come from the Mining Safety and Health Research Program at PRL. To respond to congressional guidance, NIOSH applies PRL funds only to mining safety and health issues.

Extramural activities have accounted for more than 30 percent of the Hearing Loss Research Program's overall funding since 1997. The extramural program is administered and funded through the NIOSH Office of Extramural Programs in Atlanta.

TABLE 1-1 NIOSH Hearing Loss Research Program Funding by Fiscal Year, 1997–2005

Year	Intramural	Extramural	Total
1997	$1,860,060	$ 632,405	$2,492,465
1998	$1,903,709	$ 908,010	$2,811,719
1999	$1,941,845	$1,555,768	$3,497,613
2000	$2,396,139	$1,312,928	$3,709,067
2001	$3,661,900	$1,791,830	$5,453,730
2002	$4,176,396	$2,304,960	$6,481,356
2003	$4,311,735	$1,526,709	$5,838,444
2004	$5,253,587	$1,698,416	$6,952,003
2005	$5,164,358	$2,327,408	$7,491,766

SOURCE: NIOSH, 2006a.

Facilities

Research facilities for the Hearing Loss Research Program include specialized laboratories, a mobile audiometric research facility, and instrumentation and equipment to provide comprehensive field study capabilities. The laboratories include the following facilities (NIOSH, 2005a):

- An acoustic test chamber (in Pittsburgh) is used for precision measurement of total sound emissions from large equipment. This reverberation chamber was accredited in 2005 by the National Voluntary Laboratory Accreditation Program (NVLAP) for sound power measurements in accordance with International Organization for Standardization (ISO) 3741 (ISO, 1999) and American National Standards Institute (ANSI) S12.51 (ANSI, 2002).
- Two hearing protector laboratories (one in Cincinnati and one in Pittsburgh), which were fully remodeled in 2003, include a reverberation room and computers and software to run standard hearing protector testing protocols. The laboratory in Pittsburgh is accredited by NVLAP for the measurement of real-ear attenuation of hearing protection devices in accordance with test standard ANSI 12.6-1997 R2002 (ANSI, 1997).
- Two clinical audiometric suites (one in Cincinnati and one in Pittsburgh) contain clinical audiometers (which include extended high-frequency test capability), tympanometers, otoacoustic emission measurement systems, and a hearing aid analyzer. The Cincinnati facility also includes a small audiometric test room similar to those commonly found in occupational settings. A small-animal noise exposure and test facility has been installed at the University of Cincinnati Biological Sciences Department with NIOSH funding. The university facility is equipped to test auditory evoked potentials and otoacoustic emissions in laboratory animals.
- Two anechoic chambers (a large chamber in Pittsburgh and a smaller one in Cincinnati) are used for evaluations with acoustic test fixtures. A hemi-anechoic room in Pittsburgh, which will accommodate construction equipment, was nearly complete in early 2006.
- An education and training laboratory in Cincinnati can be used to conduct studies with groups of participants examining training issues and evaluating materials, including electronic and web-based training.
- A 172 m^3 anechoic chamber at the University of Cincinnati is equipped with a 24-channel computerized data acquisition system. This chamber is used by the Hearing Loss Research Program on a collaborative basis.

Laboratory facilities also include metal-working and carpentry shops with suitable equipment and hand tools. Expert technician support is also available for these shops.

Research Administration

Intramural research projects carried out by the Hearing Loss Research Program are selected from investigator-initiated proposals. Since 2002, leadership within each NIOSH division or laboratory with activities in the program has been responsible for obtaining external peer review of proposals for assessment of their scientific quality. Selection of proposals for funding is based on considerations of scientific quality and on management review for relevance and potential for transfer to the workplace. Annual reviews for each project are carried out by the respective divisions or laboratories (NIOSH, 2005a, 2006b).

Extramural research supported by NIOSH is also investigator-initiated. Grant applications in response to Program Announcements or Requests for Applications are submitted to the Center for Scientific Review of the National Institutes of Health. This center manages the independent review of grant applications for scientific merit. Subsequent reviews for programmatic relevance are conducted by senior NIOSH scientists.

The Hearing Loss Research Program reported that it has been guided in its selection of major emphases for research by the goals described earlier in this chapter. In the past, the program's focus had largely been on developing new knowledge and increasing capacity. In the last few years and with the establishment of the NIOSH r2p ("Research to Practice") program, the focus has shifted toward consideration of the impact of the research program in the workplace (NIOSH, 2005a).

EVALUATION APPROACH

The committee was charged with reviewing the Hearing Loss Research Program to evaluate the relevance of its work to improvements in occupational safety and health and the impact that NIOSH research has had in reducing workplace illnesses and injuries. The Framework Document directs that relevance be evaluated in terms of the degree of research priority and connection to improvements in workplace protection. It identifies factors to take into account, including the frequency and severity of health outcomes and the number of people at risk, the structure of the program, and the degree of consideration of stakeholder input (see

Appendix A). The impact of the program's research is to be evaluated in terms of its contributions to worker health and safety. The evaluation is to take the form of qualitative assessments as well as the assignment of scores between 1 and 5 for the relevance and impact of the Hearing Loss Research Program's research and other activities.

The guidance in the Framework Document reflects the terminology and organization of a logic model adopted by NIOSH to characterize the steps in its work. The logic model used by the Hearing Loss Research Program appears as Figure 1-3. An examination of goals, inputs, activities, and outputs was used to assess the relevance of the program's research. End outcomes and intermediate outcomes were the principal focus for the evaluation of the impact of the program's research. External factors were taken into consideration in the evaluation. The terms used and the details of the committee's evaluation are presented in Chapter 2.

The study charge also directs the committee to review the progress that the Hearing Loss Research Program has made in identifying new research and provides the committee the opportunity to identify emerging research areas relevant to the program's mission. According to the Framework Document, the committee's identification of emerging research areas is to be done using members' expert judgment rather than a formal research needs identification effort.

THE COMMITTEE'S REPORT

The remainder of the report presents the findings from the committee's evaluation. Chapter 2 presents the committee's review of the NIOSH Hearing Loss Research Program and the ratings for the program's relevance and impact in reducing workplace injury and illness. In Chapter 3, the committee reviews the Hearing Loss Research Program's mechanisms for identifying emerging issues in occupational hearing loss and noise control and identifies issues that may warrant future attention. In Chapter 4, the committee identifies opportunities to strengthen the NIOSH Hearing Loss Research Program and increase the relevance and impact of the program's efforts.

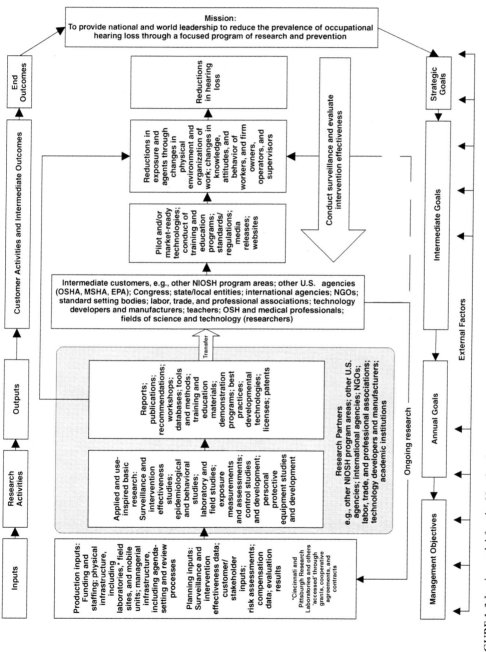

FIGURE 1-3 Logic model for the Hearing Loss Research Program. SOURCE: NIOSH, 2005a.

REFERENCES

ANSI (American National Standards Institute). 1997. ANSI S12.6. *American National Standard Methods for Measuring the Real-Ear Attenuation of Hearing Protectors*. New York: Acoustical Society of America.

American National Standards Institute. 2002. ANSI S12.51/ ISO 3741:1999. *Acoustics—Determination of Sound Power Levels of Noise Sources Using Sound Pressure—Precision Methods for Reverberation Rooms*. ANSI S12.51. New York: Acoustical Society of America.

ISO (International Organization for Standardization). 1999. ISO 3741: 1999. *Acoustics—Determination of Sound Power Levels of Noise Sources Using Sound Pressure—Precision Methods for Reverberation Rooms*. Geneva, Switzerland: ISO.

Lotz WG (NIOSH). 2006a. RE: info request. E-mail to L Joellenbeck, Institute of Medicine. May 26.

Lotz WG (NIOSH). 2006b. RE: seek technical review of figure and caption. E-mail to L Joellenbeck, Institute of Medicine. July 21.

Lotz WG (NIOSH). 2006c. RE: seek technical review of figure and caption. E-mail to L Joellenbeck, Institute of Medicine. August 1.

NIOSH (National Institute for Occupational Safety and Health). 1972. *NIOSH Criteria for a Recommended Standard: Occupational Exposure to Noise*. Pub. No. HSM 73-11001. Cincinnati, OH: NIOSH.

NIOSH. 1996. Draft Document—Criteria for a Recommended Standard Occupational Noise Exposure: Revised Criteria 1996. Noise Pollution Clearinghouse (NPC) Online Library. [Online]. Available: http://www.nonoise.org/library/niosh/criteria.htm [accessed June 14, 2006].

NIOSH. 1998. *Criteria for a Recommended Standard. Occupational Noise Exposure: Revised Criteria 1998*. DHHS (NIOSH) Pub. No. 98-126. Cincinnati, OH: NIOSH.

NIOSH. 2005a. NIOSH Hearing Loss Research Program: Overview. In: NIOSH Hearing Loss Research Program: Evidence for the National Academies' Committee to Review the NIOSH Hearing Loss Research Program. Cincinnati, OH: NIOSH. Pp. 19–40.

NIOSH. 2005b. NIOSH Overview. In: NIOSH Hearing Loss Research Program: Evidence for the National Academies' Committee to Review the NIOSH Hearing Loss Research Program. Cincinnati, OH: NIOSH. Pp. 7–17.

NIOSH. 2006a. NIOSH Hearing Loss Research Program: Intramural Projects and Budget Distribution, 1997–2005. Unpublished document provided to the Committee to Review the NIOSH Hearing Loss Research Program. Cincinnati, OH: NIOSH.

NIOSH. 2006b. NIOSH Hearing Loss Research Program: Peer Review Process for Intramural Research. Unpublished document provided to the Committee to Review the NIOSH Hearing Loss Research Program. Cincinnati, OH: NIOSH.

NIOSH. 2006c. NIOSH Hearing Loss Research Program: Research Staff Distribution by Organizational Unit. Unpublished document provided to the Committee to Review the NIOSH Hearing Loss Research Program (January 23). Cincinnati, OH: NIOSH.

NIOSH. 2006d. NIOSH Hearing Loss Research Program: Research Staff Distribution by Organizational Unit. Unpublished document provided to the Committee to Review the NIOSH Hearing Loss Research Program (January 30). Cincinnati, OH: NIOSH.

U.S. Congress. 1970. The Occupational Safety and Health Act of 1970. Public Law 91-596. Washington, DC: U.S. Congress.

2

Evaluation of the Hearing Loss Research Program

The committee was charged with reviewing the Hearing Loss Research Program of the National Institute for Occupational Safety and Health (NIOSH) to evaluate the relevance of its work to improvements in occupational safety and health and the impact that NIOSH research has had in reducing workplace illnesses and injuries. The committee's review focused on the work of the Hearing Loss Research Program primarily during the period 1996 through 2005. Information about some NIOSH activities during the first few months of 2006 was included in the committee's review. The committee followed the Framework Document developed by the Committee to Review NIOSH Research Programs (see Appendix A). This review framework directs that relevance be evaluated in terms of the degree of research priority and connection to improvements in workplace protection. It identifies factors to take into account including the frequency and severity of health outcomes and the number of people at risk, the structure of the program, and the degree of consideration of stakeholder input (see Appendix A). Research impact is to be evaluated in terms of its contributions to worker health and safety, to the extent that this can be known or surmised. This chapter presents the results of the committee's review, reported in the form of qualitative assessments of the relevance and impact of the Hearing Loss Research Program's research and other activities.

Following the guidance of the Framework Document, the committee carried out its evaluation using the terminology and organization of a logic model adopted by NIOSH to characterize the steps in its work. An examination of goals, inputs, activities, and outputs was used to assess the relevance of the program's research. End outcomes and intermediate outcomes were examined to evaluate the impact of the program's research. Illustrative examples of each of these terms as used in this report are provided in Box 2-1. The chapter's sections on relevance and impact each conclude with a summary section with the committee's overall assessment of and quantitative scores for the relevance or impact of the Hearing Loss Research Program, respectively.

The committee also identified important factors beyond the program's control that affect its activities and performance. The "external" factors with the broadest reach are discussed before the committee's assessments of the program's relevance and impact. External factors that have a more limited effect on the program's work are noted at appropriate points throughout the discussions of the program's relevance and impact.

HEARING LOSS RESEARCH PROGRAM GOALS

In 2005, NIOSH established four research goals for the Hearing Loss Research Program, under which programs of varying breadth are being pursued (see Table 2-1). NIOSH also used these four new research goals to organize the primary evidence package provided to the committee and its presentations to the committee. In turn, the committee decided to use the four goals to organize its detailed examination of the Hearing Loss Research Program, while recognizing that these research goals were not in use by the program during most of the period covered by the retrospective assessment. As noted in Chapter 1, the four research goals encompass eight of the nine research needs identified in 1998 (NIOSH, 1998a) that guided the program's work between 1998 and 2005. The 1998 goals also reflect the priority areas of "hearing loss" and "mixed exposures" that were established in conjunction with the first National Occupational Research Agenda (NORA), as well as some work related to the NORA priority areas of "control technology and personal protective equipment," "exposure assessment methods," and "intervention effectiveness research" (NIOSH, 2005d). In the sections that follow, the presentation of the committee's findings addresses both the overall program and matters concerning individual research goals.

EXTERNAL FACTORS WITH BROAD EFFECTS ON THE HEARING LOSS RESEARCH PROGRAM

The Hearing Loss Research Program operates in an environment shaped by many factors that the program cannot control. Some of these factors are so fundamental to the nature of the program that the committee found it essential to keep them in mind for all aspects of its review.

> **BOX 2-1**
> **Logic Model Terms and Examples**
>
> **Planning Inputs:** Stakeholder input, surveillance and intervention data, and risk assessments (e.g., input from Federal Advisory Committee Act panels or the National Occupational Research Agenda research partners, intramural surveillance information, Health Hazard Evaluations [HHEs]).
>
> **Production Inputs:** Intramural and extramural funding, staffing, management structure, and physical facilities.
>
> **Activities:** Efforts and work of the program, staff, grantees, and contractors (e.g., surveillance, health effects research, intervention research, health services research, information dissemination, training, and technical assistance).
>
> **Outputs:** A direct product of a NIOSH research program that is logically related to the achievement of desirable and intended outcomes (e.g., publications in peer-reviewed journals, recommendations, reports, website content, workshops and presentations, databases, educational materials, scales and methods, new technologies, patents, and technical assistance).
>
> **Intermediate Outcomes:** Related to the program's association with behaviors and changes at individual, group, and organizational levels in the workplace. An assessment of the worth of NIOSH research and its products by outside stakeholders (e.g., production of standards or regulations based in whole or in part on NIOSH research; attendance at training and education programs sponsored by other organizations; use of publications, technologies, methods, or recommendations by workers, industry, and occupational safety and health professionals in the field; and citations of NIOSH research by industry and academic scientists).
>
> **End Outcomes:** Improvements in safety and health in the workplace. Defined by measures of health and safety and of impact on processes and programs (e.g., changes related to health, including decreases in injuries, illnesses, or deaths and decreases in exposures due to research in a specific program or subprogram).
>
> **External Factors:** Actions or forces beyond NIOSH's control (e.g., by industry, labor, regulators, and other entities) with important bearing on the incorporation in the workplace of NIOSH's outputs to enhance health and safety.
>
> SOURCE: Framework Document (see Appendix A).

First, there are important limits to the ability of the NIOSH Hearing Loss Research Program to effect change in the workplace. As part of a research agency, the program is in a position to produce knowledge about workplace injuries (i.e., occupational hearing loss), noise hazards, effective hearing protection devices, and hearing conservation practices. NIOSH can also work to promote the application of this knowledge in the workplace. The actual responsibility for minimizing haz-

TABLE 2-1 Research Goals and Subgoals of the NIOSH Hearing Loss Research Program, as of February 2006

Research Goal 1: Contribute to the Development, Implementation, and Evaluation of Effective Hearing Loss Prevention Programs
  1.1. Develop criteria and recommendations for preventing occupational hearing loss
  1.2. Develop a practical guide for preventing occupational hearing loss
  1.3. Achieve a better understanding of the combined effects of continuous and impulsive noise exposures
  1.4. Develop data management tools for hearing loss prevention programs
  1.5. Develop a hearing loss simulator
  1.6. Develop a survey instrument to evaluate training effectiveness
  1.7. Develop an evaluation checklist for hearing loss prevention programs
  1.8. Develop training focused on improving hearing protection device use
  1.9. Develop a core curriculum in occupational safety and health for high school and post-secondary students that includes a module on hearing loss prevention
  1.10. Develop a hearing protector device compendium

Research Goal 2: Reduce Hearing Loss Through Interventions Targeting Personal Protective Equipment
  2.1. Develop measurement and rating methods that are representative of real-world performance of hearing protection devices
  2.2. Develop hearing protection laboratory and fit-testing methods
  2.3. Evaluate the effectiveness of hearing protection devices against impulsive noise
  2.4. Develop a hearing protection and communication system
  2.5. Develop hearing protection recommendations for noise-exposed hearing-impaired workers

Research Goal 3: Develop Engineering Controls to Reduce Noise Exposures
  3.1. Reduce noise on continuous mining machines using coated flight bars
  3.2. Reduce noise generated by roof bolting machines using wet and mist drilling
  3.3. Reduce noise exposures to construction workers using a web-based database for powered hand tools

Research Goal 4: Improve Understanding of Occupational Hearing Loss Through Surveillance and Investigation of Risk Factors
  4.1. Determine occupational noise exposure and hearing loss through national surveillance
  4.2. Characterize hearing ability in the general population through national databases
  4.3. Prevent hearing loss from impulsive noise through development of standards and instrumentation
  4.4. Improve detection and prevention of occupational hearing loss by understanding the aging component
  4.5. Prevent hearing loss by understanding the role of genetics in susceptibility to noise
  4.6. Prevent hearing loss from exposure to ototoxic chemicals alone or in combination with noise

SOURCE: NIOSH, 2005f,g,h,i.

ardous workplace noise environments and ensuring worker compliance with hearing conservation programs lies with employers, who must respond to both economic and regulatory imperatives. Some employers may resist implementation of optimum noise control measures because they are concerned, rightly or wrongly, about the possible economic impact of such measures. Authority to establish and enforce regulations concerning workplace noise exposure and hearing conservation lies with regulatory agencies such as the Occupational Safety and Health Administration (OSHA) and the Mine Safety and Health Administration (MSHA) (both of which are part of the U.S. Department of Labor). NIOSH is expected to make recommendations to these agencies, but the agencies must consider the views of other interested parties, who may have concerns that differ from those of NIOSH.

Gaining and sustaining attention to occupational hearing loss may sometimes be difficult. The condition is relatively slow to emerge, rarely requires immediate medical attention or time lost from work, and is not fatal. Longitudinal studies are often needed to test the effectiveness of new approaches to elements of hearing loss prevention programs, and such studies require willing collaboration by employers and workers. Factors such as changes in management or fiscal conditions may lead companies to withdraw from research collaborations, and turnover in the workforce may compromise the stability of study populations.

Another important consideration is that the Hearing Loss Research Program comprises a collection of activities taking place principally within five organizational units of NIOSH. Thus, the "program" is based on a matrix approach, not on being an identifiable entity in the NIOSH organization chart. In late 2005, NIOSH for the first time designated an executive staff member—Dr. Güner Gürtunca, director of the Pittsburgh Research Laboratory—to serve as the program manager of the Hearing Loss Research Program. Although Dr. Gürtunca and another senior staff member are now expected to monitor and guide the overall program effort, the matrix nature of the Hearing Loss Research Program means that the program manager does not control its budget or program portfolio. The program's funding level is the sum of the financial resources that individual NIOSH organizational units decide to apply to work on hearing loss prevention or noise control activities. The activities of the intramural program and the equivalent of about 30 professional staff members who carry it out are distributed unequally across three units located in Cincinnati and one in Pittsburgh. The selection and management of extramural projects is based in Atlanta.

The committee was also conscious of the small size of the Hearing Loss Research Program budget. During the period under review, the program's intramural funding grew from approximately $1.9 million in fiscal year (FY) 1997 to $5.2 million in FY 2005, and its extramural funding from $0.6 million to $2.3 million.

The total NIOSH budget for FY 2005 was $286 million. By comparison, the FY 2005 budget for the National Institute on Deafness and Other Communication Disorders (NIDCD) in the National Institutes of Health (NIH) was $394.3 million. Of this, research on hearing comprised more than $176 million of the extramural budget of $340.9 million, and roughly 62 percent of the $34 million budgeted for intramural research projects (Rotariu, 2006a,b).

The portfolio, staffing, and funding levels for the Hearing Loss Research Program are also shaped by congressional direction as to the amount of the NIOSH budget that is to be applied to mining safety and health. For FY 2005, the NIOSH Mining Safety and Health Research Program had a budget of $30.7 million and the equivalent of about 260 full-time staff members (NIOSH, 2006h). Approximately $3.6 million was allocated to intramural mining-focused activities (many related to underground coal mining) that are considered to be part of the Hearing Loss Research Program (NIOSH, 2006d). This work accounted for 69 percent of the Hearing Loss Research Program's intramural funding for that year and 39 percent of about 40 full-time equivalents (FTEs) (15.5 positions). Although the NIOSH mining program no longer carries a separate line item in the federal budget, Congress has directed NIOSH to maintain its current level of research effort in this area. For the Hearing Loss Research Program, this means in practical terms that the program benefits from funding supporting work related to noise control and prevention of hearing loss in the mining sector, but the program does not have discretion to redirect these funds to any of the program's other activities, which have only a small budget to address the broad goals of the program.

OTHER FACTORS AFFECTING THE HEARING LOSS RESEARCH PROGRAM

Another important factor that the committee came to understand over the course of its information gathering is the degree to which the Hearing Loss Research Program is currently undergoing change as part of NIOSH's reorganization effort in conjunction with the second decade of NORA (NIOSH, 2006g), as well as by virtue of its self-scrutiny in preparation for this committee's evaluation. As noted earlier, the program identified new research goals and named new leadership in 2005 as it prepared for this evaluation. Both the name of the program itself and the name of one of its four research goals have been modified since the evaluation began. The committee notes that the revised program name—Hearing Loss Research Program—seems to imply a narrower scope than the original name, Hearing Loss Prevention Program. While the program intends to develop a strategic plan, it has deferred that activity until the conclusion of this evaluation.

A recently increased emphasis on transferring the products of NIOSH research into workplace application is also important to note. The Office of Research and Technology Transfer was organized in 2004 to help the agency's scientific investigators better bridge the gap between concept and workplace adoption.

ASSESSMENT OF RELEVANCE

The committee recognizes that hazardous noise exposure and occupational hearing loss represent an important, and underrecognized, threat to the health and safety of U.S. workers in a variety of industries. Although recent data are not available, NIOSH has estimated that at least 4 million workers in the United States may be exposed at work to noise levels that put them at risk of hearing loss (NIOSH, 1998a). NIOSH also has estimated that 9 million workers (some of whom may be among those exposed to hazardous noise) could be at risk as a result of exposure to ototoxic chemicals (NIOSH, 2005d). At present, most hearing loss that results from occupational exposures is irreversible, and poor hearing can compromise both safety and quality of life.

In evaluating the relevance of the work done by the NIOSH Hearing Loss Research Program, the committee has assessed the degree to which the program has led and carried out research in aspects of occupational hearing loss and noise control most relevant to improvements in workplace protection.

If available, surveillance data regarding the nature and extent of the U.S. occupational hearing loss problem would form the basis for identifying priorities and targeting research. The public health approach would direct research efforts toward questions with the most potential to bring benefit to those industrial sectors or special workforce groups with the largest number of workers at risk, the highest risk of occupational hearing loss, or the greatest exposure to its risk factors. Unfortunately, no comprehensive effort to assess the extent of hearing loss among U.S. workers has been carried out for decades. In the absence of such data, both NIOSH and the evaluation committee have only information from more limited surveys, input from stakeholders, and expert judgment as a basis on which to prioritize the national and sector-specific needs in this area.

The Hearing Loss Research Program has included the extramural work[1] carried out on hearing loss as part of its program for the purposes of this evaluation. For about a decade, NIOSH has followed the NIH model for administering its

---

[1] Extramural work for the purposes of this report refers to research conducted by investigators outside NIOSH using funding from the Office of Extramural Programs. It does not include work carried out through contracts or cooperative research and development agreements (CRADAs).

extramural research program. NIOSH develops extramural programs "based on the NORA agenda, r2p [research to practice] initiatives, congressional mandates, and other emerging occupational safety and health priorities. The strategic plans of the individual NIOSH research programs will also influence extramural programs as they are developed and become more prominent in driving the research agenda" (NIOSH, 2005e). Proposals are evaluated for scientific merit by independent panels of experts, and meritorious proposals receive secondary programmatic review by a committee of senior NIOSH scientists. As the result of a "firewall" between intramural programs and the extramural funding selection process, investigators and planners within the intramural program have had little control over the selection of extramural research.

The sections that follow review the four NIOSH Hearing Loss Research Program research areas in turn, providing the committee's findings with regard to the relevance of the research completed or under way. (Committee evaluation of NIOSH's targeting of new research is discussed in Chapter 3.) At the end of the review of the four research areas, the committee discusses the relevance of the program as a whole, and provides its quantitative and qualitative evaluation.

Research Goal 1: Contribute to the Development, Implementation, and Evaluation of Effective Hearing Loss Prevention Programs

Goals and Objectives

NIOSH described three objectives for Research Goal 1: (1) providing authoritative, data-driven recommendations and guidelines; (2) developing and/or evaluating hearing loss prevention program "best practices"; and (3) developing, evaluating, and disseminating model training methods, materials, and tools. Each of these areas of effort can have an important role in either developing or synthesizing and conveying research results to minimize workplace exposure to hazardous noise. Thus, the committee found these objectives to be highly relevant to the overall aim of reducing work-related hearing loss. The activities carried out under this research goal are important to disseminating and applying information developed across the entire Hearing Loss Research Program, providing an important means of transfer to the workplace setting.

Planning and Production Inputs

Several important research planning efforts have guided the development of the agenda for this research area over the past decade. Of these, the most important have been "A Proposed National Strategy for the Prevention of Noise-

Induced Hearing Loss" in 1988 (NIOSH, 1988), which set a course for the program until *Criteria for a Recommended Standard: Occupational Noise Exposure* (NIOSH, 1998a) was issued in 1998, and the NORA hearing loss prevention initiative in 2001. Most recently, a Futures Workshop was held in April 2005 to plan for the next decade. The Hearing Loss Research Program's current objectives and work areas bear a reasonable relationship to the earlier planning activities. For example, NIOSH is clearly making efforts to address the two recommendations most closely related to this program area described in the NORA hearing loss initiative of 2001: (1) health communications research focused on training methods and (2) research to evaluate the effectiveness of compliance-driven hearing loss prevention programs. Each of the three planning efforts involved some stakeholder input, and the committee found that research in this program area reflects consistent efforts to develop working relationships with external partners in conducting activities and developing products. The committee recommends, however, that NIOSH expand the base of experts and stakeholders to whom it turns for advice and input to increase both the breadth of the disciplines involved and the depth of the scientific and programmatic expertise of these advisers.

The facilities available for this research area include two audiometric suites, an education and training laboratory, and a mobile audiometric research facility. Since 1997, the financial and staffing resources allocated to this research area have increased. The number of personnel working on projects within this program area, as represented by the number of FTEs, has increased from roughly three to almost eight, and intramural funding has grown from $498,768 to $1,132,932 (see Table 2-2). Although this growth is encouraging, the committee believes that this level of support is not adequate given the importance of and need for the work of this research area. The committee also notes that while the program area has good staffing in audiology and psychology, it lacks the epidemiologic expertise to accomplish the necessary evaluation of the effectiveness of its activities and surveillance for occupational hearing loss and hazardous noise exposure, as discussed further below.

Funding from the NIOSH extramural program expended on projects related to Research Goal 1 has fluctuated over the last decade, from a high in FY 2000 of $559,620 to a low in FY 2004 of $68,612. The funding levels reflect expenditures for from one to three ongoing projects at different times during that period.

Activities and Outputs

NIOSH has undertaken many activities categorized as part of this program area, distributed among the 10 specific areas listed in Table 2-1 and, as a result, has generated many useful publications and products for the field (NIOSH, 2005f).

TABLE 2-2 NIOSH Hearing Loss Research Program Budget and Staffing by Research Goals

	FY 1997	FY 1998	FY 1999	FY 2000
Research Goal 1: Contribute to the Development, Implementation, and Evaluation of Effective Hearing Loss Prevention Programs				
Intramural	$498,768	$443,552	$882,679	$888,571
FTEs	3.14	5.44	5.99	5.21
Extramural	$195,806	$254,171	$434,103	$559,620
Interagency Agreements	$0	$0	$0	$0
Contracts	$21,800	$214,829	$258,329	$257,680
CRADAs	None	None	None	None
Research Goal 2: Reduce Hearing Loss Through Interventions Targeting Personal Protective Equipment				
Intramural	$141,234	$0	$271,744	$339,613
FTEs	1.90	0.00	4.30	3.05
Extramural	$0	$38,897	$143,777	$0
Interagency Agreements	$0	$0	$0	$50,000
Contracts	$0	$0	$0	$0
CRADAs	None	None	None	None
Research Goal 3: Develop Engineering Controls to Reduce Noise Exposure				
Intramural	$929,618[a]	$540,419	$466,104	$862,243
FTEs	14.64[a]	6.75	8.8	11.97
Extramural	$0	$0	$0	$0
Interagency Agreements	$0	$0	$0	$100,000
Contracts	$0	$0	$0	$15,000
CRADAs	None	None	None	None
Research Goal 4: Improve Understanding of Occupational Hearing Loss Through Surveillance and Investigation of Risk Factors				
Intramural	$199,448	$164,122	$108,434	$226,573
FTEs	2.75	2.30	1.60	2.33
Extramural	$436,599	$614,942	$977,888	$753,308
Interagency Agreements	$288,888	$288,888	$288,888	$288,888
Contracts	$0	$0	$0	$0
CRADAs	HearSāf	HearSāf	HearSāf	HearSāf

NOTE: CRADA, collaborative research and development agreement; FTE, full-time equivalent.

[a]The 1997 FTE figure shown in the table, which is derived from a NIOSH database, differs from the 1997 staffing level recalled by program and budget managers (3 FTEs) (Lotz, 2006b).

SOURCE: NIOSH, 2006a,b,c,d.

FY 2001	FY 2002	FY 2003	FY 2004	FY 2005
$1,059,249	$901,939	$785,508	$1,166,467	$1,132,932
4.56	3.94	3.39	3.45	7.85
$271,729	$355,700	$110,625	$68,612	$483,270
$0	$0	$0	$0	$0
$282,680	$257,680	$264,280	$262,030	$92,851
None	None	None	None	None
$434,802	$351,846	$731,164	$875,273	$724,586
3.70	3.90	5.10	7.95	8.10
$380,196	$352,879	$0	$0	$183,679
$75,000	$50,000	$113,000	$55,000	$133,000
$0	$73,000	$0	$24,570	$0
None	None	None	None	Earphone
$1,477,267	$1,856,948	$1,753,007	$2,086,163	$2,454,984
15.02	10.3	17.23	21.1	16.27
$50,000	$215,158	$225,600	$141,400	$0
$0	$0	$0	$0	$0
$117,250	$127,250	$187,250	$191,800	$145,000
None	None	None	None	None
$653,150	$944,926	$976,153	$639,372	$453,457
4.55	6.80	7.84	6.22	3.45
$1,089,905	$1,381,223	$1,190,484	$1,488,404	$1,660,459
$288,888	$288,888	$288,888	$359,888	$359,888
$33,750	$58,750	$158,543	$142,800	$0
None	None	None	None	Impulse meter

Particularly noteworthy among these activities are the development of *Criteria for a Recommended Standard: Occupational Noise Exposure* (NIOSH, 1998a), and responses to Advanced Notices of Proposed Rulemaking from OSHA and the Department of Transportation regarding hearing conservation programs. The program also provided information to MSHA during the development of its regulation "Health Standards for Occupational Noise Exposure," issued in 1999 (see MSHA, 1999). In 1996, the Hearing Loss Research Program updated *Preventing Occupational Hearing Loss—A Practical Guide,* which had first been published in 1990, and the program is now working to repackage the contents of this publication to suit the needs of small businesses. In partnership with the Ford Motor Company and other firms, researchers developed software to support and facilitate hearing loss prevention programs. They developed a hearing loss simulator, made many of their resource materials available on the web, held workshops, and produced NIOSH publications, journal articles, book chapters, presentations, and a television appearance. The impact of this work is discussed later in this chapter.

Committee Comments on Relevance to Occupational Safety and Health

The outputs ascribed by NIOSH to this research area include some of the best-known and most frequently cited products of the Hearing Loss Research Program. Stakeholders attest to their value and usefulness in guiding professionals, employers, and workers in practices considered likely to prevent hearing loss. For example, one comment described *Criteria for a Recommended Standard* (NIOSH, 1998a) as "seminal and essential," and another wrote of the criteria document together with *Preventing Occupational Hearing Loss—A Practical Guide* (NIOSH, 1996) as having "served to push forward the state of the art in hearing loss prevention." In general, the evaluation committee found the goals and activities related to this research goal to be appropriate and highly relevant. It commends the program area for its increasing emphasis on developing the evidence base for workplace practices to reduce hearing loss, and for productive work with a variety of partners to convey research results to the shop floor.

To further enhance the program's relevance, the committee urges that more attention be directed toward evaluating the effectiveness of the education and training methods NIOSH has developed. Several evaluation studies described to the committee appear to be testing changes in workers' knowledge and attitudes about hearing conservation activities (e.g., the hazards of noise, the value of hearing protectors) rather than testing whether workers' behavior is changing (e.g., using hearing protection more often or more effectively). The committee notes favorably the assessment of the correlation between carpenters' behavioral intentions and actual hearing protector use (Stephenson, 2001; NIOSH, 2005f) and commends the intended monitoring of standard threshold shift (STS)[2] rates in shipyard workers as part of research now getting under way (NIOSH, 2005c).

The Hearing Loss Research Program materials emphasize the importance of the hierarchy of controls, giving primacy to engineering controls over other approaches to reducing harmful exposures. The committee agrees with this approach but is concerned that the NIOSH-developed training, tools, and guidelines have placed particular emphasis on administrative controls and personal protective equipment in the form of hearing protection devices, but have not emphasized the role of engineering control of noise sources. Although the "Best Practices Guide" (NIOSH, 1996) contains a chapter on engineering control and stresses its importance, the development and testing of training and materials appear to have been pursued more aggressively for considerations of workers' use of hearing protection. This may reflect the priorities exhibited by most employers for economic and other reasons. While acknowledging that industry may perceive economic obstacles, the committee urges NIOSH to consider activities that promote low-noise design and noise control engineering approaches, such as the development of education and training materials that promote the importance of and provide technical support for designing and purchasing quiet equipment.

The committee notes that many of the program's transfer efforts have focused on the construction and mining sectors, and it urges continued efforts to facilitate the transfer of prevention practices to other sectors, as planned with the repackaging of the "Practical Guide" for small businesses.

Another source of some concern for the committee is the seeming lack of appreciation and integration or application of the work carried out via the extramural program that relates to this research goal. None of the eight extramural projects funded in areas relevant to this research goal have been referenced or seemingly built upon by intramural researchers, at least as conveyed by the NIOSH evidence package. The firewall that precludes interaction between intramural researchers and extramural applicants prior to an award (NIOSH, 2005a, 2006e) should not limit productive interaction after the award is made.

Despite these caveats, the committee finds the goals, activities, and outputs of this program area in general to be addressing high-priority subject areas adequately connected to improvements in workplace protection. With limited budget and staff, the program area cannot take on all of the tasks that might seem desirable to an external committee and has done well in its selection of areas to address.

---

[2]A standard threshold shift is defined by OSHA as an average 10 dB or more loss, in one or both ears, relative to the most current baseline audiogram averaged at 2000, 3000 and 4000 Hz (29 C.F.R. 1910.95).

Research Goal 2: Reduce Hearing Loss Through Interventions Targeting Personal Protective Equipment

Goals and Objectives

For Research Goal 2, NIOSH (2005g) has identified five objectives: (1) developing measurement and rating methods that are representative of the real-world performance of hearing protection devices; (2) developing hearing protection laboratory and fit-testing methods; (3) evaluating the effectiveness of hearing protection devices against impulsive noise; (4) developing a hearing protection and communication system; and (5) developing hearing protection recommendations for noise-exposed hearing-impaired workers. The committee found that these objectives appropriately target research and development that is important to reducing occupational hearing loss. Until or unless low-noise design and noise control engineering approaches are applied universally to eliminate hazardous noise in the workplace, hearing protection devices will continue to be vital to limiting exposure to hazardous noise. All of the goals established by the Hearing Loss Research Program are of ongoing importance to the field, as discussed below.

Planning and Production Inputs

Many of the planning efforts that the Hearing Loss Research Program has engaged in since 1996 have made specific reference to research needs in the area of hearing protection devices. For example, a white paper prepared by NIOSH (1998b) in advance of a March 1998 workshop—Control of Workplace Hazards for the 21st Century: Setting the Research Agenda—which was sponsored by NIOSH, the American Industrial Hygiene Association, and the American Society of Safety Engineers, included among proposed recommendations the development of hearing protection devices that employ active noise control, active level-dependent attenuation technologies, and communication functions and the development of hearing protection devices on the basis of wearer comfort and enhanced speech understanding. (The proceedings from this workshop are still in preparation.) The 2001 NORA hearing loss initiative identified the need for characterization and field evaluation of nonlinear hearing protection devices and the need to implement new technology for improving hearing protection effectiveness. In March 2003, a U.S. Environmental Protection Agency (EPA) Workshop on Hearing Protection Devices, organized by NIOSH, explored three topics: the appropriate fitting protocol to test hearing protection devices for labeling, appropriate methods to assess performance of electronically augmented hearing protection devices, and appropriate methods for calculating the Noise Reduction Rating

(NRR) of hearing protection devices. Finally, participants in a May 2003 Best Practices Workshop on Impulsive Noise and Its Effects on Hearing, sponsored by NIOSH and the National Hearing Conservation Association (NHCA), identified research gaps that included basic research on hearing protection devices for impulsive noise and the adequacy of active noise reduction for impulsive noise. Ongoing work in this program area has largely reflected these planning inputs.

The intramural funding and personnel directed toward work in this program area increased from about $140,000 and three FTEs in 1997 to almost $725,000 and eight FTEs in 2005, with a zero budget in 1998 (see Table 2-2). Since 2000, an interagency agreement with EPA has provided additional support totaling $500,000 for research on hearing protection devices with respect to EPA labeling regulations.

Funding from the NIOSH extramural program awarded to projects contributing or related to Research Goal 2 has varied, from none in 1997, 2000, 2003, and 2004 to as much as $380,196 in FY 2001. The funding levels reflect funding for from no projects to one project.

The committee underlines the importance of continuing to support the implementation of realistic hearing protection device attenuation ratings and the development of realistic assessments of field performance. In addition, the committee encourages the agency to increase its research efforts in the less evolved areas of developing a hearing protection and communication system and developing hearing protection recommendations for noise-exposed hearing-impaired workers.

Activities and Outputs

The activities undertaken by the NIOSH Hearing Loss Research Program related to this research goal appear appropriate and of importance to improvements in hearing loss prevention, as well as responsive to the planning inputs described above. The overestimation of hearing protection device performance by the laboratory "experimenter-fit" test procedure has posed difficulties for hearing conservation professionals since the inception of the NRR concept. OSHA requires the use of the NRR despite its basis in an outdated test standard promulgated by EPA in the early 1970s (40 C.F.R. 211.206). Activities in this program area to develop technical evidence for improved measurement and labeling methods will facilitate a badly needed revision of the existing regulation that is likely to help hearing loss prevention program professionals, workers, and employers with the selection of appropriate hearing protection devices. NIOSH's inter-laboratory studies in this area have resulted in four peer-reviewed publications over 8 years, setting the stage for impacts described later in this chapter (Royster et al., 1996; Berger et al., 1998; Murphy et al., 2002, 2004). Furthermore, the role of Hearing Loss Research Program staff as technical advisers to EPA in its initiative to revamp the NRR labeling for hearing protection devices is testament to the relevance of their expertise in this program area.

Another major thrust of efforts in this program area is in developing laboratory fit-testing methods. There is an enormous need for a simple fit-testing protocol that can be used in the workplace. A protocol that can be administered onsite will provide employers and hearing loss prevention professionals with a realistic assessment of the amount of noise reduction that a worker's hearing protection device is providing. The Hearing Loss Research Program's efforts to develop and compare fit-testing methods and equipment to evaluate them have led to a new tool for researchers and developers, HPDLab. It is anticipated that HPDLab will facilitate research to improve fit-testing protocols that may ultimately be used in the field.

The program area activities and outputs related to the effectiveness of hearing protection devices against impulsive noise are of vital importance to hearing loss prevention. While research endeavors focused on understanding the energy and risk differences between impulsive and continuous noise are pursued through other program areas (see discussion of Research Goal 4), empirical evaluation of the attenuation of impulsive noise by hearing protection devices is also needed. Measuring the performance of different types of hearing protection devices in impulsive noise environments and determining the most effective types for these environments will be especially valuable to law enforcement agencies and the military. In addition, application of this information to the goal of optimizing protection during non-occupational activities with hazardous impulsive noise, such as recreational shooting, may help reduce the amount of noise-induced hearing loss from these types of activities. Thus far, outputs from these efforts have included presentations and publications, Health Hazard Evaluation (HHE) reports to two law enforcement agencies (Tubbs and Murphy, 2003; Harney et al., 2005), and an update of the hearing protection devices compendium (NIOSH, 2000a).

Activities by the Hearing Loss Research Program to develop a combined hearing protection and communication system led to the development of a prototype that has faced challenges in transferring to the workplace via private-sector development. While the committee considers the development work to have been relevant to workplace protection from hazardous noise, its failure to find real-world application demonstrates the need within NIOSH for the capabilities and assistance of the recently established Office of Research and Technology Transfer.

Finally, research begun to explore and address the needs of noise-exposed hearing-impaired workers is relevant and responsive to a research need identified in the 1998 *Criteria for a Recommended Standard: Occupational Noise Exposure* (NIOSH, 1998a). If successfully developed, practical and easy-to-enforce protocols formulated by Hearing Loss Research Program investigators that focus on how to keep such employees safe in noisy environments would be of great benefit to the occupational safety and health community.

Committee Comments on Relevance to Occupational Safety and Health

In summary, the committee finds the goals, activities, and outputs of this program area to be addressing high-priority subject areas adequately connected to improvements in workplace protection. In particular, the work of this program area in support of the revision of the test standard on which the NRR is based and in improving fit-testing methods places the Hearing Loss Research Program at the hub of current research activities concerning the selection and use of hearing protection devices.

Research Goal 3: Develop Engineering Controls to Reduce Noise Exposure

Goals and Objectives

NIOSH (2005h) described three objectives for Research Goal 3: (1) reducing noise on continuous mining machines using coated flight bars; (2) reducing noise generated by roof bolting machines using wet and mist drilling; and (3) reducing noise exposures to construction workers using a web-based database for powered hand tools. The Hearing Loss Research Program evidence materials indicate that these areas for focused research are selected by gathering and analyzing information on noise emission levels to identify the equipment used in the mining and construction industries that produces the highest noise levels and that, where engineering controls do not exist, they are designed, developed, implemented, and tested for the noise-producing equipment (NIOSH, 2005h). Although each of these objectives is appropriate and relevant to the reduction of noise in work environments, they reflect the heavy emphasis of this program area on noise controls for mining, with some additional work in the construction industry. The committee is concerned that this narrow focus neglects noise control needs in other, larger sectors such as manufacturing and small business. Further discussion of the apportionment of noise control work appears later in this section.

Planning Inputs

Circumstances in the mining sector make this an opportune time for an emphasis on noise control in mining. In 2000, MSHA's rule, Health Standards for Occupational Noise Exposure (30 C.F.R. 62), took effect. This regulation emphasizes the primacy of engineering controls for preventing noise-induced hearing loss in miners. It does not accept the use of hearing protection devices as a means of compliance with the standard (30 C.F.R. 62.130). As a result, conditions are now more favorable for the implementation of noise controls in the mining industry. In contrast, OSHA's noise exposure regulation for most industries (29 C.F.R. 1910.95) allows the use of hearing protection devices as a means of reducing exposure to hazardous noise when engineering controls are not feasible. OSHA noise exposure reduction requirements are less strong for the construction industry (29 C.F.R. 1926.52). Employers outside of mining thus have less regulatory incentive to reduce noise at the source.

Several of the planning efforts noted by the NIOSH Hearing Loss Research Program identified research needs pertaining to engineering noise controls that presumably served as planning inputs for this research area. "A Proposed National Strategy for the Prevention of Noise-Induced Hearing Loss" (NIOSH, 1988) identified as long-term regulatory objectives the development of national consensus standards to provide noise labels for new equipment and the reestablishment of the EPA program to implement provisions for product noise labeling required by the 1972 Noise Control Act. In the area of information dissemination, the proposed national strategy noted the need for development of a curriculum model to provide guidelines for buying equipment that meets federal regulations for sound power output, dissemination of guidelines showing employers how to use procurement specifications to induce manufacturers to reduce the sound power output of their machinery, and encouragement of NIOSH-supported Educational Resource Centers and other educational institutions to place more emphasis on noise control and the health effects of noise. Identified as a long-term objective was updating existing manuals for noise control products and compendia of engineering solutions in order to develop a catalog intended for health and safety practitioners who are not noise control specialists.

Criteria for a Recommended Standard: Occupational Noise Exposure (NIOSH, 1998a) names noise control as one of nine research needs to be emphasized and recommends the creation of a database of effective solutions or best practices. Similarly, the Hearing Loss Research Program's large program proposal in 2000 also identified the need to catalog and evaluate noise control techniques to create an "encyclopedia of effective noise control technology" for use by industry (NIOSH, 2000b).

The workshop Control of Workplace Hazards for the 21st Century: Setting the Research Agenda, held March 10–12, 1998, ostensibly stimulated the formulation of a national plan for research on new strategies to control existing health and safety hazards in the workplace and to anticipate and prevent emerging problems. According to the Hearing Loss Research Program evidence package, the workshop proceedings are still in final preparation to be published on the NIOSH website, so their role as a planning input to this research area is not clear and may have been limited. A white paper drafted in advance of the meeting noted tentative recommendations that included evaluating current and legacy noise control technologies, developing databases to guide selection of retrofit or new noise control technologies, conducting joint research or demonstration projects to fill technology gaps and evaluate new emerging technology, and adopting voluntary noise standards to label products used in the workplace (NIOSH, 1998b).

The Mining Research Plan was recently completed as an overall strategic plan for the NIOSH Mining Safety and Health Research Program (see NIOSH, 2006h). It identifies seven strategic goals, of which Strategic Goal 2 is "Reduce noise-induced hearing loss in the mining industry." One of four intermediate goals of this strategic goal is "developing engineering noise control technologies applicable to surface and underground mining equipment."

Finally, a Futures Workshop was held April 7–8, 2005, and cosponsored by NHCA. The summary of this workshop is not yet available, but among the research needs identified at the meeting were developing basic guidelines on engineering controls and the maintenance of those controls, providing leadership to encourage noise control education in undergraduate engineering programs, publishing available noise control solutions, developing engineering controls for small businesses, and encouraging manufacturers to provide noise labels (NIOSH, 2006f).

NIOSH notes the importance of outside review and stakeholder input to its planning and review activities. However, the committee finds that the breadth and depth of expert input drawn upon are not sufficient, either in general or for this program area in particular, which appears to be somewhat isolated from the wider noise control technical community. For example, the proposal for the NORA-funded project of 2001 included a substantial noise control engineering component entitled "Definition and Assessment of Engineering Noise Controls." The proposal was reviewed by two subject matter experts who had some concerns about it, but it is not clear that those concerns were addressed. External experts on the final review team for the overall NORA Hearing Loss Research Program proposal included no one with an industrial or product noise control background. The 2005 Futures Workshop included only six external speakers, only one of whom was from the noise control field.

NIOSH seems to have sought extensive input from the mining community on mining-related tasks, but this partnership might be broadened further, for instance with inclusion of participants from mine machinery rebuilding shops who could provide additional perspectives on incorporating noise control retrofits on old machines (since older mining machines are often rebuilt rather than discarded). It does not appear that the construction community or any other stakeholder or expert group was involved in developing the power tools database project. To the extent that industry can be persuaded to participate, its involvement may strengthen the relevance of this project. Industry participation has not been evident to date.

The committee acknowledges the challenge NIOSH faces in balancing the sometimes-competing or conflicting interests of different stakeholder groups. It is difficult to maintain a collaborative and attentive relationship with multiple stakeholders when all feel that NIOSH ought to consider their needs and status to be of the highest priority. For example, during a briefing to the committee, MSHA expressed the wish that NIOSH afford it "premier standing" as a stakeholder.

The Hearing Loss Research Program has two principal groups of stakeholders. First are the individuals and organizations in the business, labor, and public health communities outside the federal government. NIOSH needs strong relationships with these groups to accomplish its mission. They provide NIOSH with access to the workplace, ideas for programs and priorities, review of and response to research activities, and political support. Second are MSHA and OSHA, the regulatory agencies that by statute have a special relationship with NIOSH. NIOSH has responsibility for making "recommendations concerning new or improved occupational safety and health standards" that "shall immediately be forwarded to the Secretary of Labor" (U.S. Congress, 1970). Although NIOSH needs strong collaborative relationships with all of these groups, the Occupational Safety and Health Act seems to expect NIOSH to give some deference to the views of OSHA and MSHA while at the same time remaining independent, open, and responsive to other stakeholders. Thus, some accommodation to MSHA's statutory role and needs is in order, but the committee would not consider it appropriate for NIOSH to afford MSHA "premier" status.

Additional planning or information inputs from which the noise control engineering program might benefit further are the bodies of work carried out by the former Bureau of Mines and by MSHA. The Bureau of Mines was active in noise control engineering research in the 1970s, investing approximately $5 million on projects carried out by well-known and respected consultants. Although NIOSH indicated that nothing in the Bureau of Mines noise archives was worth assimilating into the current NIOSH mining noise control effort, the committee encourages further review, either for successful outcomes that can be applied or as a starting point for future research. Similarly, additional examination of work completed by MSHA might also prove valuable to NIOSH researchers and help reduce the risk of needlessly re-tackling long-standing problems.

As with the other Hearing Loss Research Program research goals, the lack of surveillance data on which to base priorities is an important gap in information available for planning regarding noise control needs in both mining and other sectors. Data cited by the program are outdated or weak, although there is an ongoing effort within the mining program to gather cross-sectional noise exposure data (Bauer and Kohler, 2000; NIOSH, 2005b). Additional strong surveillance information is needed across industrial sectors to help in the prioritization and planning of research efforts.

With regard to planning inputs, the research in this program area has been responsive to the current regulatory environment in mining and to many Hearing Loss Research Program planning documents, but has drawn upon limited relevant expertise and surveillance data in planning its activities. The committee encourages continued and improved collaborative planning among the program's intramural researchers and with regulatory agencies and increased involvement of product noise control technical experts in such planning efforts.

Production Inputs

One of the most important production inputs for this research area results from an external factor described earlier in this chapter. Funding designated by Congress for spending on mining health and safety issues cannot be redirected to health problems in other industry sectors, despite information from surveillance data, experts, or stakeholders that might support other priorities within the broader field of workplace noise control and hearing loss. Given these circumstances, the committee advocates maximizing research and development that might prove applicable outside as well as within the mining sector.

The transfer of the U.S. Bureau of Mines health and safety research to NIOSH in 1996 was followed by a substantial increase in the size of the Hearing Loss Research Program staff and its effort in noise control engineering. Intramural funding for the program area grew over the last decade to $2,454,984 in FY 2005. Over the same period, the number of personnel in terms of FTEs varied from as few as 3 in FY 1997 to more than 21 in FY 2004 (see Table 2-2).

The growth in program resources resulted primarily from two factors. Engineering noise control work, particularly in the mining sector, increased due to both external factors and program management decisions. As noted earlier, Congress directed that funding specifically support mining research. In addition, the MSHA noise regulation published in 1999 created new opportunities for partnerships and research in mining, and NIOSH management responded by reassigning researchers to increase the resources directed at the noise-induced hearing loss issue in mining. In 1997, the Hearing Loss Research Program had fewer than three employees partially focused on engineering noise control research, primarily in mining.

While the additional staff assigned to work on engineering noise control since 1997 brought expertise in mining engineering, they had little if any experience in noise control. Noise control engineering is a subspecialty of acoustical engineering and is not easily or quickly mastered. Designing robust and effective noise control engineering solutions that are not merely applications of existing strategies requires extensive engineering education and experience in the field. Source noise control (the appropriate approach for reducing noise emissions of mining and power tool equipment) is the most technically sophisticated and challenging noise control approach and one that is not likely to be implemented successfully by the simple application of concepts found in a catalog or compendium.

Although the committee commends the efforts of Hearing Loss Research Program management to increase the capabilities of its staff by supporting graduate education in noise control for some engineers, this approach can supplement but is not a substitute for recruitment of senior-level researchers with demonstrated world-class expertise in the desired focus area. The committee believes that such a step is necessary for NIOSH to play the national leadership role in industrial and product noise control stated in its mission.

Despite healthy funding for the engineering noise control efforts directed to mining, minimal funds were allocated for the power tool noise control design projects, which were undertaken as class projects supported by small grants to five universities. Although training opportunities such as these projects are important, greater investment in the work of product noise control design experts is likely to be required in order to generate robust and effective noise control designs that are acceptable to manufacturers and likely to be implemented.

Funding from the NIOSH extramural program for projects related to Research Goal 3 totaled $632,000 between FY 2001 and FY 2004 for two projects focused on active noise cancellation. These efforts (and any resulting output) do not appear to have been integrated into the work of the intramural program, even though one of the two projects involved mining equipment.

Three laboratory facilities are involved in noise emission measurement activities related to this research goal. Two of these have been able to adequately support the goals of the program, while the other has met with significant challenges. The reverberation chamber at the Pittsburgh Research Laboratory was recently accredited by the National Voluntary Laboratory Accreditation Program (NVLAP) for sound power-level determinations in accordance with ISO (International Organization for Standardization) 3741 (ISO, 1999) and ANSI (American National Standards Institute) S12.51 (ANSI, 2002). The large hemi-anechoic chamber has just been completed. The Pittsburgh noise control team indicated its intention to earn NVLAP accreditation for test procedures that will be developed for this facility.

In contrast, the hemi-anechoic chamber at the University of Cincinnati appears to be too small for some power tool measurements or to measure certain tools under load. That chamber is not NVLAP-accredited, which would be appropriate for the nature of the work being performed (where outputs would be expected to be used as the basis of third-party product noise declarations and purchase specifications, etc.). The committee has concerns about the conduct of operations at the University of Cincinnati laboratory that extend beyond accreditation, however. Data generated for the purposes of consensus standards, comparison of commercial equipment, or publicly available references for decision making should be carried out according to standardized documented procedures, with a professional level of accuracy and repeatability that can be quantified and guaranteed. It was not clear to the committee that the work met these standards.

Activities and Outputs

Projects to reduce noise on continuous mining machines and noise generated by roof bolting machines using wet and mist drilling are well under way and have generated outputs in the form of new technologies that have been described in trade journals and conference proceedings (e.g., "Noise Controls for Continuous Miners" [Kovalchik et al., 2002]). The necessary next steps to validate these technologies with full-shift noise exposure monitoring (not merely sound emission measurements) under mining conditions in a working mine are very important and highly relevant to the reduction of hearing loss in mines where they might be implemented. Should these technologies qualify as "technically achievable" according to MSHA, they are much more likely to be used, as discussed later in this chapter.

Collection of baseline power tool noise emission measurements is a necessary precursor to any product noise control design project. However, the Hearing Loss Research Program's current online power tool database is of limited value because of uncertainty in how the measurements were made (the database contains results that were obtained in accordance with a test standard that specifies unloaded conditions for some tools and loaded conditions for others, and the operating conditions are not indicated in the database) and limitations of the laboratory facility and operations where the measurements were acquired. Expert, experienced professionals should carry out this work in an NVLAP-accredited laboratory facility to ensure its quality and credibility.

NIOSH has used small contracts to involve engineering students at five universities in designing acoustical engineering controls to reduce noise from small construction tools (Hayden, 2004). Student research projects are worthwhile and important activities, but they are not a substitute for focused research by experienced professionals, whether on the NIOSH staff, at universities, or in the private sector. In supporting the small student projects, the Hearing Loss Research Program has made an effort to contribute to the development of noise control engineering capability among college students, but the program also needs more systematic plans to promote the efficient development and transfer of robust noise control designs that can be cost-effectively and realistically implemented, manufactured, and accepted by the end user community.

Several other activities related to this program area have not yet produced outputs. Among them are updates of the *Industrial Noise Control Manual* (NIOSH, 1978) and the *Compendium of Materials for Noise Control* (NIOSH, 1980). OSHA has provided $100,000 toward the effort to produce a resource with standard noise control solutions useful even for people outside the discipline of noise control (NIOSH, 2006c). Another anticipated output is the "Noise Control Guidebook for Underground Metal Mines," which was developed as part of the large NORA-funded project begun in 2001. These activities are more difficult to successfully complete than might appear because source noise control, in particular, involves expert judgments that cannot readily be reduced to generic examples for the purpose of cataloging solutions.

Finally, as far as could be ascertained, the outputs from the two extramural projects were a final report (Hodgson and Li, 2004), a master's degree thesis (Rai, 2005), and a paper (Rai et al., 2005).

Committee Comments on Relevance to Occupational Safety and Health

Although the true extent of noise-induced hearing loss in the mining sector is not well defined, the committee finds that the amount of funding that has been expended to study a very narrow range of noise control problems, in a small segment of workers, reflects an imbalance when considering the relative importance of those problems in the context of the broader industrial noise problem. Within the Hearing Loss Research Program, the focus on mining appears to shortchange other occupational sectors and pose a risk that emerging issues will not be identified.

The prioritization within this research goal reflects the results of congressional targeting of resources toward health and safety challenges in mining. Given this external factor, the committee appreciates that some of these resources are being directed to "dual-use" applications that might bring benefits to other industrial sectors, but more efforts need to be undertaken in this direction. The committee urges the program to work actively to transfer the information beyond the mining sector to other application opportunities (see Chapter 4).

The committee understands that the noise control work at the Pittsburgh facility represents a nascent effort that is still ramping up in expertise, capability, and facilities. The committee urges that senior-level expertise be recruited to provide the technical leadership needed in this important and specialized area.

Stakeholder relationships are important for providing NIOSH with input to the planning process, cooperation for workplace studies, and partnerships for the actual use of NIOSH-developed technologies or materials. Particularly in the mining sector, the Hearing Loss Research Program has done a good job of cultivating the strong relationships with stakeholders that are crucial for carrying out relevant research and development work that is validated in real-world settings. The committee urges the development of better ties to other relevant stakeholders and sources of noise control engineering expertise. In the same vein, the committee urges better awareness and integration of relevant work carried out through the extramural funding program.

In general, the committee finds the goals, activities, and outputs of this program area to be focused on subject areas of lesser priority than desirable, even taking into account the strictures limiting much of the spending to the mining sector. The targeted funding does not preclude other Hearing Loss Research Program efforts from reaping greater benefit from the work done and otherwise making a greater contribution to engineering controls for other sectors.

Research Goal 4: Improve Understanding of Occupational Hearing Loss Through Surveillance and Investigation of Risk Factors

Goals and Objectives

The six objectives described by NIOSH (2005i) for Research Goal 4 are (1) determining occupational noise exposure and hearing loss through national surveillance; (2) characterizing hearing ability in the general population through national databases; (3) preventing hearing loss from impulsive noise through development of standards and instrumentation; (4) improving detection and prevention of occupational hearing loss by understanding the aging component; (5) preventing hearing loss by understanding the role of genetics in susceptibility to noise; and (6) preventing hearing loss from exposure to ototoxic chemicals alone or in combination with noise. The committee found the main objective (establishing effective surveillance systems to monitor exposures in the workplace and the incidence of hearing loss in workers) highly relevant to reducing occupational hearing loss. If designed appropriately, such systems may also help to address questions related to the aging workforce. Research to develop standards and instrumentation for preventing hearing loss from impulsive noise and to prevent hearing loss from exposure to ototoxic chemicals is also relevant to the reduction of work-related hearing loss.

The committee had less confidence in the relevance of research objectives 2, 4, and 5 to the overall NIOSH Hearing Loss Research Program mission "to provide national and world leadership to reduce the prevalence of occupational hearing loss through a focused program of research and prevention." Although the hearing status of the general population, the role of aging in hearing loss, and the genetics of hearing loss are important research questions, the committee saw a need for NIOSH to emphasize the work-related aspect of these topics. Basic science studies pertaining to the genetic and aging aspects of hearing loss may have implications for the workplace, but they could be better supported and conducted through organizations such as NIH, with NIOSH collaborating in or building on such studies in ways that focus on workers and the workplace. Similarly, data on the hearing ability of the general population is of interest for comparison with occupational groups, but it may be more appropriate for NIOSH, with its focus on worker health, to rely more heavily on NIH or others to assemble the data for the general population. In the committee's view, the Hearing Loss Research Program should actively monitor relevant research being conducted or supported by NIH and, when appropriate, should strive to build on findings from that work.

Planning Inputs

Several planning activities and documents noted as important by the Hearing Loss Research Program have identified research needs addressed in this program area. "A Proposed National Strategy for the Prevention of Noise-Induced Hearing Loss" (NIOSH, 1988) noted short-term objectives, including analyzing data collected under the OSHA Hearing Conservation Amendment to evaluate the effectiveness of regulations. Long-term objectives included "collect[ing] hearing data for populations not exposed to occupational noise as a baseline for comparing the hearing of groups exposed to noise. Norms should be established as a function of geographic region, sex, race, age, etc." Other long-term objectives included conducting research to better define the relative hazard of different kinds of noise (impulse, impact, intermittent, etc.); determining the degree to which noise interacts with other agents in the work environment (solvents, metals, prescription drugs, etc.) to affect hearing; and describing the physiologic mechanisms associated with noise-induced hearing loss. *Criteria for a Recommended Standard: Occupational Noise Exposure* (NIOSH, 1998a) included impulsive noise, auditory effects of ototoxic chemical exposures, and exposure monitoring among the nine research needs identified.

The proposal prepared by the Hearing Loss Research Program and funded in 2001 through NORA was intended to "augment specific areas of the overall program that needed to be strengthened" (NIOSH, 2005d). The long-term objectives identified for the 5-year project included assessing the prevalence of occupational noise exposure and related hearing sensitivity, identifying critical gaps in the noise and hearing loss knowledge base, and conducting or supporting gap-filling research and developing data and recommendations to support standards and rulemaking bodies (NIOSH, 2005d).

In April 2002, the Hearing Loss Research Program together with NHCA held a Best Practices Workshop on the Combined Effects of Chemicals and Noise on Hearing (NIOSH, 2005k), with 13 outside speakers and 77 attendees. During a 2003 Best Practices Workshop on Impulsive Noise and Its Effects on Hearing (NIOSH, 2005k), participants (12 outside speakers, 43 attendees) identified five research needs for future studies: (1) instruments and standards for measurement and evaluation of impulsive sounds; (2) international consensus on descriptors for impulsive sounds and procedures for applying results from tests on animals to models for effects on humans; (3) international consensus on procedures to evaluate the effectiveness of hearing protection devices and engineering noise controls to reduce hearing loss; (4) understanding of hearing impairment resulting from exposure to impulsive sounds; and (5) damage risk criteria for impulsive sounds (Kardous et al., 2005). The 2005 Futures Workshop (with 25 NIOSH and 6 external participants) was also a part of the Hearing Loss Research Program's planning processes.

Several of the objectives for this program area were identified as research needs in planning documents or were the subject of conferences, but it is unclear from the material provided how these events have contributed to the design and implementation of current and future research activities under this program area. Although some stakeholder and outside expert input has been obtained, it appears that there are relatively small numbers of experts from outside NIOSH engaged in these planning activities. The Hearing Loss Research Program is strongly encouraged to expand its network of external advisers to better represent the current applied and basic knowledge base on noise-induced hearing loss.

Production Inputs

The budget devoted to this program area has grown considerably in the last 10 years, with the majority of these dollars channeled to extramural initiatives. Intramural funding allocated to this area varied from $108,434 to $976,153 during this time, with $453,457 budgeted for FY 2005 (see Table 2-2).

Between 1997 and 2005, an interagency agreement between the National Institute on Deafness and Other Communication Disorders and the National Center for Health Statistics provided $2.1 million to support the adult audiometry examinations that were conducted as part of the National Health and Nutrition Examination Survey (NHANES) and overseen by the Hearing Loss Research Program. NIDCD also provided $71,000 for each of FY 2004–2005 and FY 2005–2006 to support continued Hearing Loss Research Program work on the NHANES effort via a contractor.

Only a small number of FTEs at NIOSH have been engaged in Research Goal 4 activities, ranging from fewer than 2 to nearly 8 over the past decade, with the level at 3.45 in FY 2005. Given the stated major focus on surveillance and traditional epidemiologic studies, it is notable that no epidemiologist is currently involved in these activities. This is a marked contrast to other program areas in NIOSH that are known for their strong epidemiologic expertise. The committee encourages the addition of epidemiologic expertise to improve the quality of the surveillance activities within the Hearing Loss Research Program.

Extramural funding for this research area nearly quadrupled over the decade, from $436,599 in FY 1997 to $1,660,459 in FY 2005, at the same time that the number of projects funded increased from two to seven. The Hearing Loss Research Program has relied on the investigator-initiated pipeline rather than issuing requests for targeted extramural proposals.

Overall, the resources of this program area with respect to the availability of a sufficient budget, staff, and essential expertise are not adequate for its broad scope.

Activities and Outputs

As acknowledged by NIOSH, the lack of surveillance data for noise exposure or occupational hearing loss is a fundamental knowledge gap (NIOSH, 2005i). The committee views the Hearing Loss Research Program goal to "determine occupational noise exposure and hearing loss through national surveillance" as crucial and highly relevant, and in need of focused and well-designed activities to improve upon the current situation.

For many years, the Hearing Loss Research Program has been engaged in monitoring hearing in workers through health hazard evaluations, targeted industrial surveys, statewide monitoring (Michigan), and efforts to have hearing loss reported separately under the OSHA recordability standard. Some of these initiatives have involved program personnel directly in the methods and monitoring of data quality and others have not. These activities have led to outputs in the form of contributions to the *Worker Health Chartbook* (NIOSH, 2004), annual reports from a state-based surveillance program (*http://oem.msu.edu/sensor.asp*) (Michigan State University, 2004), software for more efficient use of audiometric databases, NIOSH reports, and several journal publications.

Despite these contributions, there remains a lack of reliable person-level data on the incidence of hearing loss among workers, in part because of historical approaches to hearing loss prevention that have focused on standard threshold shifts, which can occur more than once in a person. In addition, the rates of recordable standard threshold shifts now being reported by the Bureau of Labor Statistics (BLS) use FTEs for denominators. Under this model, two part-time workers may equal one FTE in the denominator and two cases of hearing loss in the numerator. As a result, data from BLS can provide only an approximation of the public health burden of occupational hearing loss, temporal trends are difficult to interpret, and the success of prevention efforts cannot be measured accurately.

In addition, the primary model in which hearing loss in an employed person is attributed exclusively to workplace noise ignores the potential contributions of exposures accrued outside of or unrelated to work, the effects of chemical exposures at work, or aging and may lead to an overestimate of the amount of occupational noise-related hearing loss. On the other hand, poor measures of noise exposure may lead to underestimates of noise-related damage to the auditory system. In the absence of good surveillance data, NIOSH has relied for many years on estimates originally dating from the 1980s and unpublished reanalyses when describing the dimensions of the hearing loss problem. Rather than repeatedly citing these unreliable estimates, the Hearing Loss Research Program needs to take concrete steps to address the lack of good numbers and published analyses.

The Hearing Loss Research Program has received feedback about its lack of surveillance efforts before. One of the reviewers of the program's large proposal for NORA funding in 2001 commented: "Unfortunately the proposed program does not include any attempt to assess the methodology for developing a surveillance system for work-related noise induced hearing loss. Such a system is crucial to assess the burden of noise-induced hearing loss, evaluate the effectiveness of hearing conservation programs, education and enforcement activity and study trends in the disease. . . . It is a major deficiency in the NIOSH noise program that no research project addresses developing methods of conducting national surveillance" (NIOSH, 2001).

Most of the Hearing Loss Research Program's recent activities to measure occupational noise exposure appear to be focused on supporting studies of specific worker groups such as miners, Washington State construction workers, those on Brazilian fishing boats, and others. Since it is not clear how generalizable these results are to other occupational settings or to the U.S. worker, it appears that surveillance of current noise exposures is inadequate. The number of workers with significant exposure to noise is simply not known, nor is there an effective mechanism for either determining change over time or identifying subgroups of workers who are at highest risk. Plans for national surveillance of workplace noise exposures were not presented.

Hearing Loss Research Program activities to help characterize hearing ability in the general population through national databases are carried out largely through partnerships. The program's audiologists have provided technical oversight of the audiometry component of NHANES as it conducts cross-sectional studies of hearing across all ages. Outputs in the form of NHANES audiometric datasets are now available to NIOSH researchers and others for analysis.

The committee is appreciative of the strategy of partnering with other agencies to ensure that high-quality data about hearing in the general population are available for the nation, and the involvement of the program's hearing professionals in the NHANES study is further recognition of their technical expertise. However, the Hearing Loss Research Program should participate in these activities only to the extent that they are also able to develop appropriate initiatives to understand the risk of occupational hearing loss.

Furthermore, the expectations from these partnerships are not necessarily appropriate. For example, the goal to use NHANES data as a non–noise-exposed reference population is not realistic. Many of the NHANES subjects are younger or older than the working population, and among those in the correct age range, many will have exposure to occupational or other noise. The committee is concerned that the sample size of non–noise-exposed individuals of working age is not sufficiently large for statistical rigor. Also, while the NHANES data will yield valuable information about the prevalence of hearing loss in the general population, it was not clear to the committee that this is germane to the primary mission of the Hearing Loss Research Program. Because of the well-known "healthy worker effect," comparisons between employed workers and the general population may not accurately measure the impact of work-related exposures on hearing health.

The Hearing Loss Research Program also hopes to gain information on the effects of aging from NHANES. NIOSH researchers assert that the data "allow for direct measurement of hearing loss due to aging in the population" (NIOSH, 2005i), but this statement reflects an inaccurate understanding of the strengths and limitations of the NHANES study design. Although the study will provide high-quality data on hearing thresholds in individuals of various ages, cross-sectional data do not provide measures of aging effects; only longitudinal data can answer that question.

The program's researchers are also providing technical assistance to studies in a small longitudinal cohort (Fels Longitudinal Study) and to the Age, Gene/Environment Susceptibility Study (AGES), a longitudinal study of Icelanders. The Fels study collected hearing thresholds and noise exposure information on children and young adults between 1977 and 1983 and will conduct repeat audiometric testing on these former youths (now adults) and their children. Without information about sample size or expected participation rates, the committee is concerned that selection and response biases will limit the utility of the results.

Furthermore, although studies of Icelanders may contribute knowledge about genetic polymorphisms important in hearing loss and aging in Iceland, it is not clear that this information will be relevant for U.S. workers. Neither of these research activities in selected samples directly addresses concerns about occupational hearing loss, or the goal of characterizing hearing ability in the general population through national surveillance.

The Hearing Loss Research Program has supported activities investigating the prevention of hearing loss from impulsive noise exposure primarily through extramural studies in experimental animal models. In addition, program personnel have evaluated existing acoustic measurement devices and standards and their limitations with regard to impulsive sounds. Current activities include developing new technology for measuring impulsive noise (in part through a cooperative research and development agreement [CRADA] with Larson-Davis, Inc.) and working toward an occupational damage risk criterion for impulsive noise exposure. Outputs have included two HHE reports, a provisional patent on an instrument for monitoring exposure to impulsive noise, a 2003 best-practices workshop on impulsive noise, and numerous peer-reviewed articles extending back 30 years.

Activities related to improving understanding of the aging component of hearing loss have been carried out primarily through a partnership with the University of Cincinnati's Department of Biological Sciences. Studies in a mouse model of early age-related hearing loss and susceptibility to noise-induced hearing loss have evaluated the impact of noise and aging on hearing and the possibility that dietary antioxidants protect the ear from early hearing loss due to aging. Outputs have included an important publication (Erway et al., 1996) and related articles, presentations, and posters, as well as a conference co-organized by the Hearing Loss Research Program entitled "The Mouse as an Instrument for Hearing Research," which was held in 2003 at the Jackson Laboratory, Bar Harbor, Maine. The Jackson Laboratory organized a follow-up meeting in 2005, with participation by a NIOSH Hearing Loss Research Program researcher.

Hearing Loss Research Program activities related to understanding the role of genetics in susceptibility to noise include the mouse model work carried out with the University of Cincinnati and AGES, the study of 10,000 Icelanders discussed above, to look for genes for hearing loss.

By far, the most well-developed research area within Research Goal 4 has been the effects of exposure to ototoxic chemicals alone or in combination with noise. The Hearing Loss Research Program has engaged in numerous studies, primarily in other countries, that demonstrate potential ototoxic effects of chemical exposures in the workplace and interactive effects of noise and chemical ototoxins. The research is novel, has been published widely in the mainstream scientific literature, and has begun to influence policy decisions. This research goal and its associated activities are highly relevant to NIOSH's mission. However, data to determine the magnitude of ototoxic chemical exposures are lacking and need to be sought. The number of U.S. workers exposed, the amount of exposure, and the risk of hearing loss associated with the exposure are not known.

As noted, extramural research represents the largest use of resources for this program area. Some of the projects have been noted above. Over the last decade, these projects have included laboratory animal studies to better predict the consequences of noise exposure, to explore basic mechanisms of noise damage to hearing, to examine interactions of chemical asphyxiants and noise in hearing loss, to apply both a statistical learning machine and a radial basis function neural network to the prediction of noise-induced hearing loss, and to explore the prevention of solvent- and noise-induced hearing loss with antioxidants. Other projects have included a cross-sectional study of hearing acuity and threshold shifts in Hispanic workers, a prospective study of hearing damage among new construction workers, a longitudinal study on effects of noise and solvents on hearing, and the development of a low-cost miniature personal noise dosimeter. All of these efforts represent investigator-initiated research. With the exception of work in the area of ototoxicity, there has been limited effort by intramural researchers to build on the extramural research. To bring more focus to high-priority research topics for occupational hearing loss, the committee recommends that the program consider generating Requests for Applications and Program Announcements to help focus extramural researchers on issues highly relevant to the mission of the Hearing Loss Research Program (see Chapter 4).

Committee Comments on Relevance to Occupational Safety and Health

This program area is the smallest by far of the four research areas in terms of funding and staffing, representing less than 10 percent of the Hearing Loss Research Program intramural budget and FTEs in FY 2005. Nevertheless, Research Goal 4 has the broadest and perhaps the most difficult program objectives to achieve. Taking into account the scale and strengths of the Hearing Loss Research Program, the highest priority should be given to areas that are fundamental to addressing occupational hearing loss. The distinction is captured in the two titles that the Hearing Loss Research Program has used for this goal. The original name was "Contribute to reductions in hearing loss through the understanding of causative mechanisms." More recently, the program has adopted the current name, "Improve understanding of occupational hearing loss through surveillance and investigation of risk factors." The committee sees the name change as appropriate, but notes that the emphasis of the work also needs to change to reflect the importance of both surveillance and occupational hearing loss (as opposed to hearing loss in general).

The committee sees the research goals of determining occupational noise exposure and hearing loss through national surveillance, preventing hearing loss from impulsive noise through development of standards and instrumentation, and preventing hearing loss from exposure to ototoxic chemicals as highly relevant to reductions in workplace noise or hearing loss. The challenges described earlier of carrying out effective surveillance in occupational hearing loss and noise exposure necessitate the investment of financial resources and epidemiologic expertise commensurate with the importance of surveillance data to setting priorities for the whole program. The committee recommends a better alignment of allocated resources with the scope of the challenges.

The committee views the objectives and activities related to understanding the aging and genetic components of hearing loss and assessing hearing loss in the general population as less relevant to preventing occupational hearing loss. Although there are important questions to be answered about the relationships between hearing loss, aging, and genetics, the current projects reflect a diffusion of the mission from worker safety to basic science questions, which are less relevant for NIOSH and could be better supported or conducted by other organizations such as NIH. Data that will be generated from audiometric surveys of the general population will be of interest, but cannot meet unrealistic expectations for their usefulness for comparison with occupational populations.

It appeared to the committee that most projects undertaken as part of this research area developed not from strategic planning efforts, but from opportunities offered and initiated by others. While appreciating the leveraging of limited resources that this has represented, the committee recommends an approach to planning based more on Hearing Loss Research Program priorities, for both its intramural and its extramural research. With limited resources, it is important to select opportunities that will directly address the goals of the Hearing Loss Research Program.

In contrast to activities and outputs in other Hearing Loss Research Program areas, there has been less emphasis in this program area on transferring knowledge to key stakeholders. For this research area, the key stakeholders are the scientific community. Analyses of databases that have been influential in determining policy have remained unpublished (Franks, 1996, 1997a,b) and criticisms have gone unanswered (Clark, 1997; Dobie, 1997). The committee emphasizes the importance of publication in peer-reviewed journals as a means to enhance the credibility of the work as well as to communicate findings to other scientists and contribute to the scientific knowledge base.

The work carried out as part of this research goal includes efforts, particularly related to understanding ototoxins, that are highly relevant to preventing occupational hearing loss. However, the committee finds the goals and activities of this program area to include several lesser-priority subject areas only indirectly connected to workplace protection, while giving insufficient effort and resources to the fundamental needs in surveillance for occupational hearing loss and hazardous noise exposures. Particularly because of its limited resources, it is important that the Hearing Loss Research Program focus on the priorities most closely related to its mission.

OVERALL EVALUATION OF THE RELEVANCE OF THE HEARING LOSS RESEARCH PROGRAM

To arrive at its qualitative evaluation and quantitative score for the relevance of the NIOSH Hearing Loss Research Program, the committee strove to step back from its part-by-part examination of the program as presented above and consider the program as a whole. Doing so raises several issues discussed at the start of this chapter that pertain to the program considered in its entirety: (1) the program is not conceived and planned as a whole, but at present is the sum of parts contributed by several divisions and a laboratory within NIOSH; (2) the largest portion of the program in terms of financial resources and staffing is designated for study of hearing loss prevention in mining, and these resources cannot be redirected to hearing loss needs in other industrial sectors; and (3) the entire program is funded at only $7.5 million, a level dwarfed by the scale of the challenge it faces in helping to facilitate the reduction of work-related hearing loss for the nation.

Acknowledging the factors above, the committee considered various ways to arrive at a single number to convey a measure of the relevance of the total program. The Framework Document (Appendix A) that guided the committee's evaluation does not prescribe a method to arrive at an overall, quantitative score from the qualitative evaluations of separate program areas. As was apparent from the review of the relevance of each of the four research areas within the total program, the committee found considerable variation in relevance across the components of the program as presented. The committee deliberated carefully about how the various research areas should be weighted, either explicitly or implicitly, in arriving at a final score. In contrast to the approach described later for arriving at a score regarding the *impact* of the work of the Hearing Loss Research Program, the committee chose to weight all of the program's activities nearly equally in contemplating the *relevance* of the work.

The charge to the committee requires an assessment of the relevance of the program's activities to the improvement of occupational safety and health. The

Framework Document ties relevance scores to the priority of subject areas and to the degree of connection to improvements in workplace protection (Appendix A). What determines "high priority"? The public health approach to prioritization relies on surveillance data to identify populations or sectors where the greatest good can be accomplished with the least effort. The Hearing Loss Research Program acknowledges the absence of current data on the incidence of occupational hearing loss or prevalence of hazardous noise exposure in the workplace, citing in its stead data that are old or weak (or, at best, unpublished) to justify the importance of this occupational health problem.

Lacking these data, one of the most important influences on the Hearing Loss Research Program in its prioritization process has been input from stakeholders, including partners from industry, labor, regulatory agencies, and professional associations. In both the NORA process and other planning activities, NIOSH has involved stakeholders in an effort to discern and prioritize research needs. Stakeholders and partners were involved in the development of "A Proposed National Strategy for the Prevention of Noise-Induced Hearing Loss" (NIOSH, 1988), which guided research in the Hearing Loss Research Program for a decade, and in identification of the research needs articulated in *Criteria for a Recommended Standard: Occupational Noise Exposure* (NIOSH, 1998a). Mining partners such as the United Mineworkers of America, the Bituminous Coal Operators Association, the National Mining Association, Joy Mining Machinery, MSHA, and others make up "the Noise Partnership" that facilitates research on noise reduction of mining equipment (NIOSH, 2005j). These partners also provided important input to the development of the Mining Research Plan, in which "Reduce noise-induced hearing loss in the mining industry" is one of seven strategic goals (Lotz, 2006a). Most recently, the Hearing Loss Research Program involved a limited number of external participants in a Futures Workshop to help set research priorities.

Given the importance of stakeholders to the Hearing Loss Research Program's priority setting, the committee has concerns about the size of the community to which NIOSH turns for input, and it urges an effort to draw on a broader and deeper set of people from both scientific and other communities to help make this an outstanding program (see Chapter 4).

An assessment of relevance must take into account the input and interests of stakeholders. Stakeholder involvement and input into NIOSH research prioritization were most apparent and laudable in the area of development, implementation, and evaluation of hearing loss prevention programs, at least as manifested by participation in conferences and workshops. The committee received input from a variety of stakeholders in the course of its information gathering (see Chapter 1 and Appendix B), including representatives from labor, industry, regulatory agencies, professional organizations, and academic researchers. With some exceptions noted elsewhere in this report, stakeholders (many of whom have partnered or collaborated with the Hearing Loss Research Program) expressed positive opinions about the relevance and appropriateness of the program's research efforts.

The committee notes that despite the Hearing Loss Research Program's intentions to develop a strategic plan in the future, it is evident—and even noted candidly in the evidence package (NIOSH, 2005d)—that management of the program over the last decade has taken place more by opportunity than by objective. For a research organization as small as the Hearing Loss Research Program, "management by objective" will be difficult. NIOSH depends on employers to enable access to appropriate study populations; therefore the program may not have the opportunity to study some of the most hazardous settings, and the continuity of the work that is undertaken can be interrupted with changes in management or lower-level staff (e.g., a project with Ford [NIOSH, 2005f]). In addition, by virtue of its role as a research rather than a regulatory organization, the program may be able to influence, but cannot set, the agenda for development of recommended regulations. Management by opportunity has also had its merits—in the past the program has skillfully leveraged its limited resources by collaborating with others.

The committee urges a balance. The Hearing Loss Research Program should seize opportunities in the context of a plan that keeps its efforts focused on the most relevant work. Using the limited surveillance information available, information from stakeholders, and its members' expert judgment, the committee found that the Hearing Loss Research Program mission and four main research goals were highly relevant to the overall aim of reducing occupational hearing loss. However, the committee considered some of the objectives or activities within these broad research areas to be less relevant to the goal of reducing work-related hearing loss.

On the basis of its review, the committee has assigned a score of 3 for the relevance of the NIOSH Hearing Loss Research Program. According to the Framework Document, a score of 3 indicates that research focuses on lesser priorities and is loosely or only indirectly connected to workplace protection (see Box 2-2).

ASSESSMENT OF IMPACT

End Outcomes

In considering the impact of the work by the NIOSH Hearing Loss Research Program, it is necessary to recognize that NIOSH and its research programs can never be expected to impose the changes in the workplace or in the behavior of workers that are necessary to reduce or prevent adverse health outcomes. What the program can be expected to do is to contribute knowledge about hazards and the

> **BOX 2-2**
> **Scale for Rating Program Relevance**
>
> 5 = Research is in highest-priority subject areas and highly relevant to improvements in workplace protection; research results in, and NIOSH is engaged in, transfer activities at a significant level (highest rating).
> 4 = Research is in high-priority subject area and adequately connected to improvements in workplace protection; research results in, and NIOSH is engaged in, transfer activities.
> 3 = Research focuses on lesser priorities and is loosely or only indirectly connected to workplace protection; NIOSH is not significantly involved in transfer activities.
> 2 = Research program is not well integrated or well focused on priorities and is not clearly connected to workplace protection and inadequately connected to transfer activities.
> 1 = Research in the research program is an ad hoc collection of projects, is not integrated into a program, and is not likely to improve workplace safety or health.

prevention of adverse outcomes and to promote plausible, evidence-based, risk-reducing actions by others, including regulatory authorities, equipment manufacturers, employers, and workers. Such actions constitute intermediate outcomes, and the committee relied on them in making its assessment of the impact of the Hearing Loss Research Program.

Nevertheless, it would be desirable to be able to consider the impact of a NIOSH research program on the basis of data on a relevant work-related health outcome—an end outcome—such as occupational hearing loss. Another somewhat less direct indicator, but defined as an end outcome in the committee's evaluation guidance, could be evidence of changes in exposure to a workplace hazard such as excessive noise. Where application of work by NIOSH was evident, a decline in the incidence or severity of the health outcome or a reduction in a hazardous exposure might suggest a beneficial impact from NIOSH's work, whereas no change or an increased incidence or exposure might suggest a lack of impact.

In trying to make judgments about the impact of work done by the Hearing Loss Research Program, however, the committee was unable to consider evidence for any of the four research goals that changes have occurred in end outcomes related to occupational hearing loss. As noted, there is a general lack of surveillance data on occupational hearing loss and noise exposures for U.S. workers during the past decade.

Even if surveillance data were available, it would be necessary to understand whether changes in these outcome measures were related to the application of products from the Hearing Loss Research Program or were the result of other factors that were producing changes in the workplace or the workforce that influence levels of noise exposure or hearing loss. For example, a decline in average noise exposure among manufacturing workers might result from adoption of NIOSH recommendations for better engineering controls for noise, but it also might reflect an increase in the proportion of the manufacturing workforce engaged in work that is inherently less noisy rather than a reduction in noise levels in high-noise environments.

Data on hearing loss and noise exposures in specific workplaces or for smaller populations of workers are also scarce. A suggestive indication of a NIOSH contribution to a reduction in occupational hearing loss came from observational data from Ford Motor Company, where a model hearing loss prevention program was developed and implemented as a collaborative effort among Ford, the United Automobile Workers, and NIOSH. From 1990 through 1998, the percentage of annual audiometric tests showing an STS declined from almost 7 percent to slightly less than 4 percent (Lick, 2001; NIOSH, 2005f). However, additional information about STS levels for the years before the project and about the workplace and the workforce before and during the project period would be needed to reach conclusions about the contribution of the model hearing loss prevention program.

Few longitudinal research studies have been conducted to test the potential impact on hearing loss or noise exposure of the application of NIOSH research products either under controlled conditions or in routine work environments. Research studies can be designed to allow for the analysis of health outcomes as well as the workplace and workforce. Because occupational hearing loss typically develops over a period of years, longitudinal studies are valuable, but they are time consuming and may be expensive. Turnover in the workforce may make it difficult to maintain a stable and adequately sized study population over the course of a study. The studies also are vulnerable to conditions in the business environment, which may discourage employers from agreeing to participate or may lead them to withdraw once a study has begun.

Intermediate Outcomes

Given the lack of data on changes in the end outcomes of occupational hearing loss and noise exposure, the committee instead based much of its assessment of the impact of the NIOSH Hearing Loss Research Program on evidence that the program's research products have been put to use beyond NIOSH in ways that have the potential to influence the workplace. Evidence of these intermediate outcomes was available, in varying degrees, for all four research goals. In some instances, the committee also considered the potential for future impact from Hearing Loss Research Program publications and other program outputs that were not yet associated with intermediate outcomes.

Research Goal 1: Contribute to the Development, Implementation, and Evaluation of Effective Hearing Loss Prevention Programs

The committee saw substantial evidence that NIOSH activities related to this research goal have been adopted or adapted for use by employers, labor, audiology and occupational safety and health professionals, and government agencies. Publications and other products of the Hearing Loss Research Program that are related to Research Goal 1 have influenced health and safety regulations, the policies of professional organizations, and the education and training of hearing health professionals and members of the workforce.

Regulations The Occupational Safety and Health Act of 1970 (U.S. Congress, 1970), which called for the creation of NIOSH, authorized the agency to establish recommended occupational safety and health standards for noise control and hearing loss prevention. The NIOSH Hearing Loss Research Program has offered such recommendations most recently with *Criteria for a Recommended Standard: Occupational Noise Exposure* (NIOSH, 1998a). The authority to establish and enforce regulations regarding occupational safety and health standards rests with other agencies, particularly OSHA and MSHA. During the period under review, both of these regulatory agencies proposed or adopted new regulations related to occupational hearing loss, and the NIOSH Hearing Loss Research Program contributed technical assistance and public comments that reflected the 1998 recommendations. Since 2002, NIOSH has also provided technical assistance in the development of hearing loss prevention regulations to other agencies, including the Department of Transportation, Department of the Interior, Federal Aviation Administration, and California Division of Occupational Safety and Health (Cal/OSHA).

The Hearing Loss Research program also made recommendations to OSHA about definitions of recordable occupational hearing loss and the need to record and monitor hearing loss separately from other occupational injuries and illnesses. A formal rule-making process, initiated by OSHA in 1996, resulted in the adoption of a revised criterion for recordable hearing loss and a new reporting form (the OSHA 300 log; 29 C.F.R. 1904.10) that provides for listing hearing loss separately from other occupational injuries and illnesses. These changes were implemented in 2004. The national data on occupational hearing loss that will become available as a result are a welcome new resource but will not meet the need for reliable person-level data on the incidence of occupational hearing loss.

Although the NIOSH Hearing Loss Research Program's recommendations for an 85 dBA exposure limit and a 3-dB exchange rate have not been adopted in OSHA or MSHA regulations, officials from these agencies informed the committee that NIOSH recommendations and comments are essential information for their rule-making processes. The committee concluded that failure to adopt specific NIOSH recommendations in federal regulations should not be interpreted to mean that NIOSH's work has had no impact on those regulations. OSHA and MSHA rule making must respond to many different, and often competing, interests and perspectives on the costs and benefits of noise exposure standards. It is not possible to know whether federal regulations would offer their current level of protection for workers if contributions from the NIOSH Hearing Loss Research Program had not been available. The committee commends NIOSH for continuing to bring its recommendations to the attention of OSHA and other agencies responsible for regulating noise exposure of U.S. workers.

Also of note is that the NIOSH recommendations are consistent with and in some cases have probably influenced the noise exposure standards adopted by the Department of Defense (DoD, 2004), individual branches of the U.S. military (e.g., Department of the Army, 1998), the National Aeronautics and Space Administration (NASA, 2006), and other countries. The U.S. Army also refers to NIOSH research on ototoxicity in a fact sheet (USACHPPM, 2003) and has incorporated consideration of exposure to ototoxins in its hearing conservation program (Department of the Army, 1998). Stakeholder comments to the committee also noted that some employers have adopted the NIOSH recommendations even though they are not required by federal regulations.

Voluntary and professional standards Influential standards and guidelines concerning the measurement of noise and noise hazards are developed not only by government agencies but also by national and international standards organizations. Personnel from the Hearing Loss Research Program serve as expert members of working groups established by committees of these voluntary standard-setting organizations.

As reported by the Hearing Loss Research Program (NIOSH, 2005f), the program's recommendations concerning impulsive noise were influential in the adoption of revisions to the international (ISO, 1990) and U.S. (ANSI, 1996) standards on noise exposure and noise-induced hearing loss. These standards have incorporated provisions that permit adding 5 dB to the measured time- and A-weighted sound level (L_{eq}) values when impulsive noises are a substantial component of a noise exposure. However, participants in the best-practices workshop on impulsive noise (convened by NIOSH and NHCA) suggested that there is no scientific evidence to justify a specific adjustment factor (Kardous et al., 2005).

Various professional organizations have incorporated NIOSH recommendations or drawn on the results of research conducted or supported by the NIOSH Hearing Loss Research Program in official statements for their members. For example, the American Academy of Audiology's 2003 position statement "Preventing Noise-Induced Occupational Hearing Loss" (AAA, 2003) bases its description of "best practices" for hearing loss prevention programs on NIOSH (1996) guidance and its recommendations for an 85 dBA noise exposure limit and a 3-dB exchange rate on the NIOSH (1998a) criteria document. In addition, researchers from NIOSH served on the task force that developed the statement. Similarly, the American Speech–Language–Hearing Association (ASHA, 2004) drew on NIOSH publications and research from the Hearing Loss Research Program for its technical report "The Audiologist's Role in Occupational Hearing Conservation and Hearing Loss Prevention Programs."

The American Industrial Hygiene Association includes NIOSH recommendations from 1998 in its standard reference publication *The Noise Manual* (Berger et al., 2000), and the American College of Occupational and Environmental Medicine (ACOEM, 2002) cites NIOSH-sponsored research in its evidence-based position statement "Noise-Induced Hearing Loss." Comments by stakeholders in Australia, France, and Sweden illustrated familiarity with NIOSH recommendations and publications in the international community as well.

Commercial products and product guides The committee also found evidence that work related to Research Goal 1 was being used to guide the selection and use of hearing protection devices. *The Hearing Protector Device Compendium* originally appeared in print form in 1976, with subsequent updates through 1994 (Franks et al., 1994). It is now available to users in an electronic form online (*http://www2a.cdc.gov/hp-devices/hp_srchpg01.asp*) (NIOSH, 2000a). The compendium is being used or cited by employers, unions, universities, vendors, other government agencies, and professional associations. Comments submitted to the committee from stakeholders confirm awareness of this resource in a variety of settings. Noted specifically was the usefulness of the online version of the Hearing Protector Compendium as an aid in the selection of appropriate hearing protection devices and as a tool for researchers. The impact of the compendium is also reflected in the decision by some manufacturers to voluntarily submit subject-fit data on the noise attenuation of their products. The committee strongly encourages the Hearing Loss Research Program to conduct the planned evaluation study to learn more about the effect of use of the compendium on the selection of hearing protection devices and the prevention of occupational hearing loss.

Through a CRADA, the Hearing Loss Research Program worked with software and industry partners to contribute to the development of revised software for the management and analysis of data collected in hearing conservation programs. Transfer of this product to the workplace has been accomplished, with the software being marketed in a commercial product, the HearSaf 2000 Suite. The Hearing Loss Research Program reports that this software has been used in collaborative projects with General Motors and the United Automobile Workers.

Education and training Products of the Hearing Loss Research Program are used widely in education and training programs for occupational safety and health professionals. *Preventing Occupational Hearing Loss—A Practical Guide* (NIOSH, 1996) has been widely adopted for use by occupational audiology graduate courses. In addition, the Council for Accreditation in Occupational Hearing Conservation (CAOHC) covers NIOSH recommendations alongside OSHA- and MSHA-required policies in its Course Director Workshops and Professional Supervisor Courses. The *Hearing Conservation Manual* produced by CAOHC (Suter, 2002) includes a version of the *Practical Guide's* program evaluation checklist and has an appendix that compares OSHA compliance criteria with NIOSH recommendations. This manual is used in many CAOHC-approved courses that certify occupational hearing conservationists (approximately 24,000 nurses, technicians, occupational physicians, and allied personnel) in the United States.

The Hearing Loss Research Program also provided the committee with materials and encouraging statements about the impact of training programs on the use and effectiveness of hearing protection devices for groups of carpenters and a request by the U.S. Navy to test the training with shipyard workers. Workers who received either form of training were observed to use hearing protection more than workers who had not received the training and to have improved attenuation from their hearing protectors (NIOSH, 2005f). The committee is encouraged to see the plans for additional study of the effectiveness of these training approaches for shipyard workers. Prospective studies are needed to determine if workers who receive training can maintain the improved fit and attenuation of their hearing protection and if they develop less hearing loss than untrained workers in a comparable noise environment.

The potential impact of establishing the effectiveness of these training approaches includes direct benefits not only to individual workers, but also to the evaluation of hearing loss prevention programs. If better training in use of hearing protection devices can be shown to have a strong association with the prevention of hearing loss, it may be possible to make more timely assessments of the effectiveness of hearing loss prevention programs by evaluating worker training in the use of hearing protectors and by fit-testing workers' hearing protectors.

Other products related to Research Goal 1 are intended for both professional and lay audiences. A hearing loss simulator developed by the Hearing Loss Research Program and designed for use on a personal computer is being used with workers and in training programs for health and safety professionals by other government agencies (including MSHA), manufacturers and vendors of hearing protection devices, universities, and professional associations. A small NIOSH study of miners and support staff ($n = 89$) was described as having found that exposure to the simulator produced significant increases in knowledge of hearing loss prevention and intentions to take more effective hearing conservation actions. The materials provided to the committee did not, however, describe how long the workers' hearing conservation intentions persisted after exposure to the simulator (NIOSH, 2005f). To make a better determination of the potential impact of the hearing loss simulator among workers, the committee emphasizes the need for further studies that examine changes in the actual use of hearing protection and adherence to other practices that reduce noise exposure.

The Hearing Loss Research Program has also contributed a component on hearing loss prevention to a broader NIOSH activity to develop an occupational safety curriculum for high schools and technical training programs. The Hearing Loss Research Program reported (NIOSH, 2005f) that the curriculum was formally endorsed by the State Directors of Career Technical Education in November 2005 and will be adopted and integrated into Career Clusters programming in every state once final revisions are completed. The U.S. Job Corps is also expected to adopt the completed curriculum, and the OSHA Training Institute has already used the hearing loss prevention part of the curriculum.

NIOSH is involved in WISE EARS!® (*http://www.nidcd.nih.gov/health/wise/*) (NIDCD, 2006), a national health education campaign on noise hazards and prevention of hearing loss. The Hearing Loss Research Program is a partner in the program with the NIDCD, and NIOSH aided in building a diverse coalition of more than 80 supporting organizations in the public and private sectors. NIOSH also contributed to the development, testing, and dissemination of the campaign's messages and materials. The WISE EARS! fact sheet on work-related hearing loss is a NIOSH product and hosted on the website of the NIOSH Hearing Loss Research Program (*http://www.cdc.gov/niosh/topics/noise/abouthlp/workerhl.html*). Participation in WISE EARS! also may help bring the Hearing Loss Research Program and its products to the attention of the broad audience represented by the members of the coalition. Evaluation of the WISE EARS! program will help the Hearing Loss Research Program and other participants learn whether it is reaching its intended audiences or influencing hearing health outcomes.

The committee also notes the potentially subtle but valuable impact that the Hearing Loss Research Program may be having through Research Goal 1 and its promotion of the term "hearing loss prevention program" as an alternative to "hearing conservation program." Reframing the goal of these activities as prevention of hearing loss may help underscore the importance of early and continued attention to workers' exposure to noise hazards. This change in terminology was explicitly noted in a technical report from the American Speech–Language–Hearing Association (ASHA, 2004). The committee found, however, that within NIOSH, recent HHE reports continue to refer to hearing conservation programs (e.g., Cook et al., 2001; Snyder and Nemhauser, 2003; Tubbs, 2003; Achutan et al., 2004; Methner et al., 2004), which may represent missed opportunities to reinforce the prevention message.

Dissemination of information and materials Many of the materials developed by the Hearing Loss Research Program in conjunction with work related to Research Goal 1 are available from NIOSH online. Evidence that other organizations are repackaging and distributing these materials signals endorsement of their value by others and may serve to influence wider audiences than distribution by NIOSH alone. Information from the *Practical Guide* (NIOSH, 1996) has been distributed through the National Safety Council publications *Today's Supervisor* and *Safeworker*. In 2005, NIOSH began working with OSHA and NHCA to develop print and electronic materials based on the *Practical Guide* that can meet the needs of small businesses.

Hearing Loss Research Program staff have contributed to the dissemination of information and materials developed for this research goal through publications, including articles in peer-reviewed journals, book chapters, and papers in conference proceedings; through presentations at conferences and workshops; and by working directly with interested parties in other government agencies, industry, labor, and the occupational health and safety community. The committee was also given information about the dissemination of electronic and print materials through NIOSH. Since 2003, the electronic version of the 1998 criteria document on the NIOSH website received more than 21,000 visits, and from January 2003 to June 2005, the *Practical Guide* (NIOSH, 1996) received more than 13,000 visits. Since 2000, more than 1,100 organizations and individuals have requested copies of the printed versions of these documents. Nearly 10,000 print copies of the *Practical Guide* (NIOSH, 1996) were sent in response to these requests, and almost 15,000 copies were distributed at meetings of the NHCA, American Academy of Audiology, American Association of Occupational Health Nurses, National Safety Congress, American Industrial Hygiene Association, Ohio Safety Congress, and Allied Construction Industries and at other hearing health, service provider, and trade meetings (NIOSH, 2005f).

Although providing information to potential users is a crucial step, the committee cautions that publications and data on distribution of materials do not demonstrate use of the material provided. Furthermore, the Hearing Loss Research Program does not appear to have established criteria by which to judge whether the demand for its materials is appropriate or should be higher overall or in specific target audiences.

Summary assessment Information provided by the Hearing Loss Research Program and comments from many stakeholders offer strong endorsement of the contributions made to efforts to reduce occupational hearing loss through work related to Research Goal 1—contribute to the development, implementation, and evaluation of effective hearing loss prevention programs.

Nevertheless, the committee found that the Hearing Loss Research Program has not paid enough attention to evaluating the effectiveness of recommendations, training programs, and other products in terms of reducing the incidence or severity of occupational hearing loss or achieving important intermediate outcomes of sustained improvement in use of hearing protection or management of hearing loss prevention programs. Evaluation based on changes in knowledge, attitudes, or behavioral intentions is appropriate but not sufficient. Furthermore, some researchers (e.g., Clark, 1997; Dobie, 1997) have suggested that the data and analyses underlying some of the program's recommendations should receive further scrutiny from the scientific community.

The committee is cognizant of factors that may be hindering the ability of the Hearing Loss Research Program to assess or improve the impact of its work related to Research Goal 1. Testing the effectiveness of hearing loss prevention measures requires collaboration with employers and workers, but as noted elsewhere in this report, hearing loss may be given relatively low priority in some settings. The program has worked successfully with various partners, but it has also experienced loss of access to data and study populations with staff changes at work sites.

Research Goal 2: Reduce Hearing Loss Through Interventions Targeting Personal Protective Equipment

The impact of the work of the Hearing Loss Research Program related to Research Goal 2 can be seen in substantial contributions to improving measurement of the fit and performance of hearing protection devices, with the results of that work influencing regulations and standards nationally and internationally. Work concerning hearing protection against impulsive noise and the hearing protection needs of workers with existing hearing impairments has been less extensive but is generating guidance for federal agencies.

Regulations, recommendations, and voluntary standards Use of hearing protection devices is central to efforts to prevent noise-induced hearing loss among U.S. workers. Regulations issued by EPA (40 C.F.R. 211.206) specify that the noise attenuation offered by hearing protection devices—the Noise Reduction Rating—must be determined by a method specified in ANSI S3.19-1974 (ANSI, 1974). Work dating from the late 1970s by Hearing Loss Research Program staff and others has shown that this method of measuring noise attenuation seriously overstates the protection that most wearers receive (see NIOSH, 1998a). In particular, the NRR, which is derived from laboratory tests of devices that are fit by experimenters, overestimates noise reduction compared with reductions obtained when hearing protection devices are fit by test subjects. Hearing Loss Research Program scientists also showed that subject-fit protocols reduced inter-laboratory variability in noise reduction compared to other fit methods. One impact of this work on hearing protection devices could be said to be evident in the Hearing Loss Research Program itself. The NIOSH (1998a) recommendations for a noise standard incorporated information on the limitations of the NRR and presented alternative approaches for judging the noise attenuation obtained with hearing protection devices.

The Hearing Loss Research Program has also influenced the work of professional and voluntary standards organizations. NIOSH staff participated in an NHCA task force that recommended use of subject-fit protocols for testing hearing protection (Royster, 1995). Staff members have also served on working groups of the ANSI S12 committee, which develops voluntary standards for hearing protector testing and rating. A standard adopted in 1997 by that committee (ANSI, 1997) includes provisions for subject fit, a testing protocol, and sample sizes that are supported by citations of four publications to which NIOSH staff contributed. In 2003 and 2005, Hearing Loss Research Program staff served as U.S. delegates to related technical committees of the International Organization for Standardization and aided in developing a draft standard based on ANSI S12.6-1997 that was circulated for consideration in 2005.

The findings that the NRR overstates noise reduction have also influenced actions by U.S. regulatory agencies. The findings were a factor in the MSHA ruling in 1999 that miners' noise exposures are to be determined without adjustments for the use of hearing protection devices (30 C.F.R. 62.110). The OSHA hearing conservation regulations, which date from the 1980s, continue to give credit for the attenuation of hearing protection devices in determining workers' daily noise doses, but reference to newer hearing protector testing protocols in the 1997 ANSI standard have been incorporated into the OSHA (1999) Technical Manual for the agency's compliance safety and health officers (see *http://www.osha.gov/dts/osta/otm/noise/hcp/hp_labeling.html*).

Work is being done to develop revised EPA regulations on the NRR. EPA officials confirmed for the committee that Hearing Loss Research Program staff helped stimulate current consideration of revisions to the regulations and have for many years provided essential technical support to EPA concerning these regulations. The technical assistance provided to EPA has included assessing hearing protector technology and product effectiveness, developing and evaluating testing standards, and performing analyses for new rating schemes. Hearing Loss Research Program staff also aided EPA by developing, managing, and participating in the analysis of results from a six-laboratory study to compare two methods for testing hearing protector attenuation.

Technology development and transfer The work related to Research Goal 2 has achieved a degree of impact through the development of a new technology that is being used beyond NIOSH. A laboratory-based system for testing the attenuation of hearing protectors, HPDLab, was developed in collaboration with a commercial partner, Howard Leight Industries. This system meets the requirements of both ANSI S3.19 and ANSI S12.6 (ANSI, 1974, 1997). The system has been installed at the NIOSH facilities in Cincinnati and Pittsburgh and at the Howard Leight Industries laboratory in San Diego. The Hearing Loss Research Program reported that Howard Leight has participated in a NIOSH-sponsored study to test the system in multiple laboratories. The system is also being used at Howard Leight to test the firm's products. An Army research laboratory and a commercial firm are installing the system for use in developing communication systems.

The Hearing Loss Research Program estimated that the cost of the HPDLab system is about $15,000, which is less than one-fifth the cost of systems developed commercially, and it does not require the customization necessary with a commercially developed system. Wider adoption of HPDLab may substantially reduce the cost of developing new hearing protector testing laboratories, but the committee does not have a basis for estimating the need for such facilities.

The committee is also aware that the NIOSH testing facility in Cincinnati is not certified by NVLAP. Because the Hearing Loss Research Program is an important contributor to work on fit and performance testing for hearing protection devices, the committee concluded that it is vital for the Cincinnati facility to achieve NVLAP certification. Achieving this status will help ensure the credibility of hearing protection device testing results from the NIOSH facility.

In the early 1990s, the Hearing Loss Research Program developed and patented a device, called EarTalk, to provide electronic communication capability in combination with hearing protection. One firm has licensed the technology, but more recent efforts to move the technology into commercial production have not been successful. In a 2002 test of a prototype EarTalk system at Wright-Patterson

Air Force Base, the system did not achieve a level of speech intelligibility comparable to more expensive systems used by the military. In 2004, the Hearing Loss Research Program received a small amount of funding through NIOSH's then-new r2p program for a transfer effort, but the program's commercial partner ultimately withdrew, citing other competing priorities.

Although the impact of EarTalk has been limited, the committee emphasizes that it is inevitable and reasonable to expect that some worthwhile efforts may not achieve intended outcomes or may achieve them over a longer time frame than the current review. However, it is also important for the Hearing Loss Research Program to ensure that its approach to commercialization efforts is based on sound business principles and is adequately supported.

Needs of workers with hearing impairment Workers who have existing sensorineural hearing impairments need to protect their remaining hearing ability and may need protection that is compatible with the use of hearing aids. Laboratory and field testing is being done to develop a protocol to guide the selection of hearing protection devices that maximize speech intelligibility for hearing-impaired workers while providing appropriate noise exposure reduction. The Hearing Loss Research Program reported that it has used the early results of this work to offer consultations and presentations to provide guidance to OSHA, MSHA, employers, and professional organizations on managing the hearing protection needs of employees with hearing impairments.

Health Hazard Evaluations Hearing Loss Research Program staff participate in NIOSH HHEs that investigate potential hazards to hearing. These investigations present opportunities to convey the program's research findings and recommendations on best practices to specific employers and groups of workers. HHE investigations of firearms training facilities for law enforcement personnel (Tubbs and Murphy, 2003; Harney et al., 2005) included consideration of hearing protection against exposures to impulsive noise, an issue being addressed under Research Goal 2. The Hearing Loss Research Program reported to the committee that the U.S. Citizenship and Immigration Service (formerly the Immigration and Naturalization Service) of the Department of Homeland Security and Oak Ridge National Laboratory in the Department of Energy are implementing NIOSH recommendations on selection and use of hearing protection devices for personnel exposed to hazardous impulsive noise.

Summary assessment In its review of the work related to Research Goal 2, the committee found that the Hearing Loss Research Program has made important contributions to increasing knowledge about the real-world performance of hearing protection devices, improving the methods and tools for assessing hearing protector attenuation, and encouraging relevant agencies and organizations to modify noise regulations and other guidance concerning hearing protector attenuation. The ability of the Hearing Loss Research Program to help constituents in the field of hearing protection device regulation reach consensus around ANSI S12.6-1997 has been especially noteworthy. The committee suspects that participation by Hearing Loss Research Program staff not only in intramural research but also in collaborations with other agencies and with academic scientists, hearing protector manufacturers, employers, and workers adds to the impact of the program in ways that are difficult to trace.

Work related to Research Goal 2 that is still maturing has the potential to have substantial impact on hearing loss prevention practices and the health of noise-exposed workers. The committee notes in particular the efforts to develop practical methods of testing hearing protector fit in the workplace and to characterize the effectiveness of hearing protection devices against impulsive noise.

Research Goal 3: Develop Engineering Controls to Reduce Noise Exposure

The impact of the work of the Hearing Loss Research Program related to Research Goal 3 is evident primarily in areas related to mining, particularly the development of quieter equipment for underground coal mining and contributions to MSHA's regulatory activities. Although some noise control developments related to mining could be applied in the construction industry, the Hearing Loss Research Program's work related to Research Goal 3 appears to have had little impact in other industrial sectors to date.

Technology development and transfer Work related to Research Goal 3 has resulted in the development of modifications to two products that are now being manufactured and used in coal mines. To accomplish the development and application of these products, the Hearing Loss Research Program participated in a collaborative effort with labor, mine operators, equipment manufacturers, and MSHA.

One product is a chain conveyor with coated flight bars for continuous mining machines. MSHA identified this product as a "promising" noise control technology in a 2004 Program Information Bulletin (McKinney et al., 2004). The chain conveyor with coated flight bars that the Hearing Loss Research Program helped develop is currently being manufactured and sold by Joy Manufacturing, Inc. This manufacturer produces more than 80 percent of the continuous mining machines in the United States, which suggests that the coated flight bar technology for chain conveyors is accessible to many coal mine operators. The Hearing Loss Research

Program reported that the technology is in use at two coal mines, but no data were provided on any measured changes in noise exposures of workers in those mines.

The other noise control technology cited by the Hearing Loss Research Program is the application of wet or mist drilling systems to roof bolting machines that are used in underground coal mines. Roof bolting machines equipped for wet drilling are currently available from J.H. Fletcher and Co., the leading U.S. manufacturer of roof bolting machines. Hearing Loss Research Program researchers verified the effectiveness of a mist system sold as a retrofit for roof bolting machines. MSHA classified wet drilling (where compatible with the geology and mining method) as a "technologically achievable" noise control and mist drilling as a promising control (McKinney et al., 2004).

MSHA defines a technologically achievable noise control as one that contributes (alone or in combination with other controls) to a 3-dBA reduction in noise exposure (McKinney et al., 2004). The committee was informed that wet and mist drilling systems are currently in use in six mines (Matetic, 2006). Any change in miners' noise exposures in these mines was not described in the materials provided to the committee.

Regulations and standards MSHA officials (Seiler and Pon, 2006) informed the committee that NIOSH provides essential research support to MSHA's regulatory and enforcement activities. Specific contributions by NIOSH related to engineering controls have included providing consultation and support during the rulemaking process for the 1999 MSHA noise standard (30 C.F.R. Part 62) on the hierarchy of hazard controls and the feasibility of engineering noise controls. Also noted were NIOSH contributions to the MSHA policy statement "Technologically Achievable, Administratively Achievable, and Promising Noise Controls" (McKinney et al., 2004).

With the MSHA noise standard's emphasis on engineering controls to meet noise exposure limits, there is a strong basis for a linkage between MSHA and work related to the Hearing Loss Research Program's Research Goal 3. By contrast, the Hearing Loss Research Program's work on engineering controls appears to have a weaker connection to OSHA. The OSHA noise standard dates from the early 1980s and, while stating a preference for engineering solutions to excess noise exposure, allows for reliance on hearing protection devices to meet exposure limits. Since the mid-1990s, OSHA has taken some preliminary steps toward additional regulation of noise exposure and hearing conservation in the construction industry. An OSHA representative (Maddux, 2006) reported that the Hearing Loss Research Program is supporting this early regulatory work by providing information on noise levels of equipment at construction sites that OSHA will use in refining risk assessments. The committee noted, however, that only one NIOSH publication on noise control, which dates from 1978, is included in the references on the "Controls" page of the Noise and Hearing Conservation section of the OSHA website (OSHA, 2005; see *http://www.osha.gov/SLTC/noisehearingconservation/hazards_solutions.html*).

Work related to Research Goal 3 also appears to be contributing to the development of voluntary standards on construction noise. The database developed by the Hearing Loss Research Program on sound levels generated by powered hand tools (see *http://www.cdc.gov/niosh/topics/noise/workplacesolutions/toolsDatabase.html*) was used as an information resource by drafters of the proposed ANSI S10.46 construction noise standard.

Powered hand tool database   The powered hand tool database project has the potential to provide information that could assist employers, workers, and the public in the selection of quiet equipment. During July and August 2005, the website for the powered tool database received 633 visits, but it is not possible to determine whether or how these visitors used the information. This work may not be well recognized by the power tool industry. The website for the Power Tool Institute, whose members include major manufacturers of powered hand tools and whose mission includes promoting safe use of these tools, includes no references to NIOSH or the powered tool database (see *http://www.powertoolinstitute.com/links.html*).

The committee is concerned that the testing of the power tools was done in a university facility that lacks NVLAP accreditation. The small size of the testing laboratory limited the size of tools that could be tested, and the facility's lack of NVLAP accreditation may undermine the credibility of test results. In particular, relying on a group of unrelated contractors, assisted by students, to conduct tests in an unaccredited facility for what appears to be intended to serve as a national reference database struck the committee as inappropriate and offering little basis for seeking to enhance the impact of the database.

The committee is also concerned that the searchable version of the database does not provide users with complete information about the conditions under which tools were tested (under load or unloaded) and that therefore the information on sound levels produced may be misleading. Without knowing whether the reported sound pressure levels are for loaded or unloaded operating conditions, users of the database may make inaccurate calculations of noise doses or hearing protection device requirements. This situation suggests the possibility that the database in its original form could have an adverse impact on hearing loss prevention. In discussions with committee members, Hearing Loss Research Program staff agreed that the operating condition under which the tools were tested should be added as a field in the searchable online database. The committee notes that the database had not been updated at the time this report was being completed.

Training Despite its concern about the database of sound levels of powered hand tools, the committee recognizes that development of the database provided an opportunity for the Hearing Loss Research Program to collaborate with the University of Cincinnati and to have an impact through expanding training resources and experience for researchers. The university's acoustics laboratory was upgraded, and a small number of engineering researchers gained training and hands-on experience in sound power level testing.

In a separate activity, engineering students at five universities participated in projects to identify noise sources and develop new noise controls or apply existing controls to reduce overall noise emissions from powered tools. Two papers produced as a result of these projects were recognized by the Institute of Noise Control Engineering as "student paper of the year" in 2003 and 2004.

The Hearing Loss Research Program also reported that enrollment in a University of Cincinnati acoustics class had increased by 10 to 15 students since the program's partnership with the university. The committee cautions that increased enrollment in a single class at a single university constitutes a very modest impact for the Hearing Loss Research Program.

Health Hazard Evaluations HHEs are generally a response to concerns about hazards in a specific workplace and therefore have a limited potential for impact. They do not provide a basis for planned efforts to address noise control needs, but in a few instances (e.g., Harney et al., 2005), HHE reports have presented an opportunity to identify ways in which employers can reduce noise generation and transmission in a given workplace. Because NIOSH does not routinely revisit HHE sites, it is not possible to determine the extent to which suggested noise control actions were implemented.

Summary assessment For Research Goal 3, the committee found that the Hearing Loss Research Program is engaged in a narrow set of activities on engineering noise controls and that these activities have had a limited impact and may have limited prospects for future impact. With the larger share of the work related to Research Goal 3 taking place at the Pittsburgh Research Laboratory, the focus is on engineering noise controls for mining. Mining equipment incorporating the results of two projects pursued by Hearing Loss Research Program staff and their collaborators outside NIOSH is being produced by manufacturers and is in use in at least a small number of underground coal mines. The program has also made contributions to efforts by MSHA to identify technologically feasible and promising noise controls for use in mining.

The Hearing Loss Research Program's work on engineering noise controls appears to have had little focus or impact on industrial sectors beyond mining. Only 2 of the 38 stakeholders who submitted comments to the committee cited engineering controls in their remarks about the program's work, outputs, or impact. One of them specifically noted the apparently low impact of the work, attributing this to lack of resources. Given the focus on mining in Pittsburgh, it seems likely that engineering noise control work related to other industries would be done through the program's Cincinnati facility, where staffing, facilities, funding, and leadership for such work have been minimal.

Development of the database on noise emission levels of powered hand tools has the potential to contribute information to users of these tools, but it makes no contribution to the development of engineering noise controls for them, either in the design of the products or in their use. The committee is concerned about the Hearing Loss Research Program's approach to creating the powered hand tool database. The work for what appears to be intended as a national reference database was done in an unaccredited facility without the benefit of a strong quality control program or organizational structure governing the operations of the laboratory. In addition, the database, as originally published, is incomplete because it lacks information about the operating conditions under which the tools were tested.

The student projects to design noise control solutions for powered tools provided an opportunity for a few students to be introduced to noise control engineering. However, this training experience represents little near-term contribution on the part of the Hearing Loss Research Program to the development of robust and manufacturable noise control solutions for these widely used tools.

The committee is aware that external factors have had some bearing on the Hearing Loss Research Program's noise control engineering efforts. With the promulgation of the MSHA noise standard in 1999, engineering noise control gained primacy over hearing protection devices for preventing occupational hearing loss in mine workers. This change prompted increased interest in the mining community in collaborating to develop engineering controls for mining equipment noise. The emphasis on mining in the Hearing Loss Research Program's work on engineering noise controls is reinforced by the availability of funding within NIOSH for work targeted specifically to mining safety and health.

By contrast with the MSHA standard, the OSHA noise standard allows for greater reliance on hearing protection devices to meet noise exposure limits. As a result, in industries other than mining, the regulatory and economic incentives have been insufficient to stimulate much interest in developing engineering noise controls. OSHA representatives confirmed to the committee that the lack of regulatory pressure for engineering noise controls in the manufacturing and construction sectors, which are under OSHA's jurisdiction, helps make it difficult for the

Hearing Loss Research Program to successfully transfer engineering controls, some of which may originate in work related to mining, to a broader range of workplaces and equipment manufacturers.

Research Goal 4: Improve Understanding of Occupational Hearing Loss Through Surveillance and Investigation of Risk Factors

The Hearing Loss Research Program's work related to Research Goal 4 has been directed in large part to data gathering, epidemiologic studies, and studies using laboratory animals to investigate the causative mechanisms of hearing loss. Over the past decade an increasing proportion of the work related to this research goal has been performed extramurally. Scientific advances typically accrue slowly from work of this sort, especially from studies in laboratory animals. Even with a high degree of success in determining the biological mechanisms through which hearing loss arises, contributions to the desired end outcomes of reductions in the incidence or severity of occupational hearing loss are likely to occur through processes that may be long, unpredictable, and not under the control of NIOSH. In assessing the impact of work related to this research goal, the committee considered contributions to the knowledge base to be important intermediate outcomes.

Scientific knowledge Through both intramural and extramural work, the Hearing Loss Research Program has produced new knowledge about the complex factors that may contribute to occupational hearing loss. The program has conducted or supported novel studies to document the potential ototoxic effects of chemical exposures in the workplace and the interactive effects of chemical ototoxins and noise, to assess the differential effects of impulsive and continuous noise, and to investigate the genetic factors contributing to susceptibility to noise-induced hearing loss using mouse models. The NIOSH evidence package noted that various papers reporting on this research are being cited in the research literature, and numerous comments received from stakeholders acknowledged the program's contribution to scientific knowledge about hearing. Although the direct impact of these studies cannot be measured in terms of "ears saved," the studies are part of long-term endeavors that contribute to improvements in human hearing health.

Surveillance Surveillance is a major focus for this research goal, and the Hearing Loss Research Program has contributed to some advances. During the period under review, the program worked with OSHA to establish new procedures for reporting occupational injuries and illnesses that provide for identifying recordable cases of hearing loss separately from other conditions. The reporting change was implemented in 2004. The new OSHA reporting requirements for hearing loss are enabling BLS to provide annual data on the number of cases of recordable hearing loss in various industrial sectors. This is a welcome step toward documenting, on a national level, the magnitude of the hearing health problem among workers. The data will also provide a means to monitor patterns of workers' hearing losses over time.

Previously, data on occupational hearing loss were being reported on a regular basis only by the State of Michigan (see Rosenman and Panasuk, 2004; see also NIOSH, 2004). Beginning in 1992, the Hearing Loss Research Program provided technical and financial support to Michigan to establish a case ascertainment system for noise-induced hearing loss through the Sentinel Event Notification System for Occupational Risks (SENSOR). The Michigan program includes referral assistance for companies that do not have their own hearing conservation programs. The Michigan data are a mix of reports of standard threshold shifts and hearing tests showing thresholds that meet specific criteria; the data come from employers' hearing conservation programs and reports from audiologists and otolaryngologists.

The newly available national data and the Michigan data are welcome information, but the epidemiologic value of both datasets is somewhat diminished by their case definitions and denominators. These data collection systems do not make use of traditional epidemiologic definitions of hearing loss and methods to capture person-level data to measure the true incidence of hearing loss in workers. Another concern is that the proportion of hearing loss cases that are identified may vary among industries. The committee commends the Hearing Loss Research Program for its success in raising awareness of the need to document the occurrence of hearing loss in workers, but the committee also emphasizes that it is essential for the program to have epidemiologic expertise fully integrated into its work on surveillance to help maximize the utility of the data collected.

Standards and guidelines The Hearing Loss Research Program's work on ototoxic chemicals is contributing to wider attention to potential ototoxic hazards of workplace exposure to certain chemicals, alone or in combination with noise. As noted in conjunction with Research Goal 1, the U.S. Army refers to NIOSH research on ototoxicity in a fact sheet (USACHPPM, 2003) and has incorporated consideration of exposure to ototoxins in its hearing conservation program (Department of the Army, 1998). The Hearing Loss Research Program has also worked with various organizations to help prepare guidelines on best practices related to ototoxic substances. For example, the American Conference of Governmental Industrial Hygienists (ACGIH) notes ototoxic chemical hazards in the noise section of its *Threshold Limit Values and Biological Exposure Indices* (ACGIH, 2003). Occupational ototoxic hazards are addressed outside the United States in worker compensation legislation in Australia and Brazil and in worker health and safety standards, such as a 2003 directive issued by the European Parliament and the Council of the European Union (2003). Explicit links to NIOSH and the Hearing Loss Research Program are not necessarily evident, but with the extensive publication record of program researchers, it seems reasonable to credit them with some influence on these developments.

Summary assessment The Hearing Loss Research Program cannot be expected to demonstrate the impact of the work conducted as part of Research Goal 4 on the basis of outcomes such as reductions in the incidence rate, numbers of cases, or severity of occupational hearing loss. The committee does, however, consider contributions that the work makes to the knowledge base on occupational hearing loss to be important intermediate outcomes. These contributions are essential steps along the pathway to effective public policies and improved public health outcomes.

The program's work on ototoxicity is widely cited by other researchers and is reflected in the hearing conservation policies of some organizations. Support for OSHA's implementation in 2004 of separate reporting of recordable occupational hearing loss has contributed to generating at least a minimal form of national surveillance data, which NIOSH and other researchers will be able to use to learn more about contemporary patterns of occupational hearing loss. The committee considers it very likely that application of knowledge generated by the program about the effects of chemical exposures and impulsive noise on hearing will lead to greater awareness of these effects and to improved worker health and safety in the future. For the program's work on genetic and age-related aspects of hearing loss, however, some contribution to basic knowledge regarding hearing health is possible, but work being done in these areas seems unlikely to contribute to knowledge regarding noise exposure and hearing loss among workers.

OVERALL EVALUATION OF THE IMPACT OF THE HEARING LOSS RESEARCH PROGRAM

As it did with its assessment of the relevance of the Hearing Loss Research Program, the committee's evaluation of impact reflects consideration of the program as a whole as well as its components, as represented by the four research goals. It was not possible to assess the program's impact on the basis of changes in the incidence or severity of occupational hearing loss or in noise exposure experienced by workers. Indeed, the lack of such data on these end outcomes is one of the major challenges of the field. The committee turned to what it considered intermediate outcomes to make its assessment of impact.

In making its assessment of the impact of the Hearing Loss Research Program, the committee considered how to combine the varied evidence of the program's impact. The conclusion reached was that the committee's rating should rest primarily on the degree to which evidence of positive impact could be observed. Areas of limited impact were not allowed to detract on an equally weighted basis from more successful efforts.

The committee found that the Hearing Loss Research Program has made contributions through publication of findings from intra- and extramural research in the peer-reviewed scientific literature, collaborative development of technologies for application in the workplace, collection and publication of resource materials for technical and lay audiences, development and delivery of educational programs, participation in the development of various national and international voluntary standards concerning noise and hearing loss, development of recommendations on noise exposure limits and hearing loss prevention practices, and consultation and collaboration with regulatory agencies.

It is clear to the committee that many of the program's work products have been adapted or adopted for use by business, labor, and occupational health professionals. Examples include adoption by the U.S. Army of the 1998 NIOSH recommendations for an 85 dBA 8-hour time-weighted average as constituting a 100 percent daily noise dose and use of a 3-dB exchange rate for determining trade-offs in the level and duration of noise exposure, and acceptance of the NIOSH recommendation for a 3-dB exchange rate and an 85-dB exposure limit by major professional organizations. Stakeholders reported widespread use of *Preventing Occupational Hearing Loss—A Practical Guide* (NIOSH, 1996) and the hearing protector compendium.

The committee found that the Hearing Loss Research Program has made important contributions to increasing knowledge about the real-world performance of hearing protection devices, improving the methods and tools for assessing hearing protector attenuation, and encouraging relevant agencies and organizations to modify regulations and other guidance concerning hearing protector attenuation.

The program provided support for establishing the feasibility of MSHA's listed engineering noise controls, contributed to rule making requiring noise control as the primary focus of occupational hearing loss prevention in mines, and contributed to international standards and heightened awareness by some U.S. organizations of the ototoxicity of several chemicals used widely in industry. In addition, the program encouraged the implementation by OSHA of new procedures for reporting occupational hearing loss on the OSHA 300 log, which will provide some basis for monitoring national patterns of workplace hearing loss. The program's participation in health hazard evaluations presents an opportunity to inform workers and employers about workplace noise hazards and to make recommendations for corrective steps that are based on the program's work in various areas, but in practice, the impact of these site-specific reviews is likely to be limited.

The committee sees the program as being, despite its small size, a unique and essential resource in efforts to protect workers' hearing. With no authority to establish or enforce regulations concerning workplace noise exposure and hearing conservation, some of the program's impact must be achieved through activities such as consultation with regulatory agencies, principally OSHA, MSHA, and EPA, and with employers, workers, equipment manufacturers, and occupational safety and health professionals. The impact of contributions in the form of formal and informal consultation, advice, and recommendations may be difficult to document but should not be discounted.

Nevertheless, the committee found that the Hearing Loss Research Program has not given sufficient attention to consideration of performance criteria related to intermediate or end outcomes. Developing such criteria could aid the program in identifying desired forms of impact, targeting efforts toward achieving those outcomes, and assessing progress. A related concern is the need for more attention to evaluation of the effectiveness of the program's activities and the view that some of the evaluation efforts that are being made could be more useful if they were based on end outcomes, such as reducing the incidence or severity of occupational hearing loss, or on achieving important intermediate outcomes, such as sustained improvement in the use of hearing protection or in the management of hearing loss prevention programs. Evaluation based on changes in knowledge, attitudes, or behavioral intentions is not sufficient.

The committee is also concerned that too little attention has been given to developing data on the incidence and severity of occupational hearing loss and the levels and extent of noise exposure among workers. Such data are essential for determining the most meaningful impacts of the work of the Hearing Loss Research Program. Developing and maintaining surveillance systems present substantial challenges, but well-designed longitudinal research studies could provide not only valuable descriptive information on noise exposure and hearing loss but also the opportunity to test the effectiveness of recommended hearing loss prevention measures.

The program may also be missing the opportunity to help build a stronger scientific basis for aspects of occupational hearing loss prevention. With a few notable exceptions, researchers in the Hearing Loss Research Program have made only limited contributions to the peer-reviewed research literature. Presentations and other kinds of publications are important contributions, but they cannot take the place of formal documentation of research results. Timely publication of research results and conference proceedings helps keep the wider scientific community informed about the program's work and encourages other researchers to test and build on findings from the NIOSH program. Relying on unpublished analyses as a foundation for important policy recommendations may, in the long run, weaken the credibility of those recommendations.

The program's narrow set of activities in engineering noise controls appears to have had a limited impact, mostly in mining, and may have limited prospects for future impact, especially in other industrial sectors. Development of the database on noise emission levels of powered hand tools is a source of concern because of the lack of rigor in the laboratory operations and the lack of attention to the content and performance of the online database. The committee also considers the student projects to design noise controls as offering little prospect for impact on noise exposures. Furthermore, work regarding genetic and age-related aspects of hearing loss is likely to make some contribution to basic knowledge in these areas, but will not readily contribute to knowledge regarding noise exposure and hearing loss among workers.

On the basis of its review, the committee has assigned the NIOSH Hearing Loss Research Program a score of 4 for impact, notwithstanding significant shortcomings in some aspects of the program. This score reflects a judgment that the Hearing Loss Research Program has made a moderate contribution on the basis of well-accepted intermediate outcomes, has generated important new knowledge, and is engaged in transfer activities (see Box 2-3). This score reflects the committee's assessment that the program has had identifiable and worthwhile impact that should not be discounted because of lesser degrees of impact from some aspects of the program.

BOX 2-3
Scale for Rating Program Impact

5 = Research program has made a major contribution to worker health and safety on the basis of end outcomes or well-accepted intermediate outcomes.

4 = Research program has made a moderate contribution on the basis of end outcomes or well-accepted intermediate outcomes; research program generated important new knowledge and is engaged in transfer activities, but well-accepted intermediate outcomes or end outcomes have not been documented.

3 = Research program activities or outputs are going on and are likely to produce improvements in worker health and safety (with explanation of why not rated higher).

2 = Research program activities or outputs are going on and may result in new knowledge or technology, but only limited application is expected.

1 = Research activities and outputs are NOT likely to have any application.

NA = Impact cannot be assessed; program is not mature enough.

REFERENCES

AAA (American Academy of Audiology). 2003. Position Statement: Preventing Noise-Induced Occupational Hearing Loss. Reston, VA: AAA.

Achutan C, Tubbs RL, Habes DJ. 2004. NIOSH Health Hazard Evaluation Report, HETA 2004-0014-2929: Navajo Agricultural Products Industry, Farmington, New Mexico. Cincinnati, OH: NIOSH.

ACGIH (American Conference of Governmental Industrial Hygienists). 2003. *Threshold Limit Values for Chemical Substances and Physical Agents and Biological Exposure Indices.* Cincinnati, OH: ACGIH.

ACOEM (American College of Occupational and Environmental Medicine). 2002. ACOEM Evidence-based Statement: Noise-Induced Hearing Loss. Chicago, IL: ACOEM.

ANSI (American National Standards Institute). 1974. ANSI S3.19-1974. *Method for the Measurement of Real-Ear Protection of Hearing Protectors and Physical Attenuation of Earmuffs.* New York: Acoustical Society of America.

ANSI. 1996. ANSI S3.44. *Determination of Occupational Noise Exposure and Estimation of Noise-Induced Hearing Impairment.* New York: Acoustical Society of America.

ANSI. 1997. ANSI S12.6. *American National Standard Methods for Measuring the Real-Ear Attenuation of Hearing Protectors.* New York: Acoustical Society of America.

ANSI. 2002. ANSI S12.51/ ISO 3741:1999. *Acoustics—Determination of Sound Power Levels of Noise Sources Using Sound Pressure—Precision Methods for Reverberation Rooms.* ANSI S12.51. New York: Acoustical Society of America.

ASHA (American Speech–Language–Hearing Association). 2004. The Audiologist's Role in Occupational Hearing Conservation and Hearing Loss Prevention Programs. Technical Report. Rockville, MD: ASHA.

Bauer ER, Kohler JL. 2000. Cross-sectional survey of noise exposure in the mining industry. In: Bockosh G, Karmis M, Langton J, McCarter MK, Rowe B, eds. *Proceedings of the 31st Annual Institute of Mining Health, Safety and Research.* Blacksburg: Virginia Polytechnic Institute and State University. Pp. 17–30.

Berger EH, Franks JR, Behar A, Casali JG, Dixon-Ernst C, Kieper RW, Merry CJ, Mozo BT, Nixon CW, Ohlin D, Royster JD, Royster LH. 1998. Development of a new standard laboratory protocol for estimating the field attenuation of hearing protection devices. Part III. The validity of using subject-fit data. *Journal of the Acoustical Society of America* 103(2):665–672.

Berger EH, Royster LH, Royster JD, Driscoll DO, Layne M, eds. 2000. *The Noise Manual,* 5th ed. Akron, OH: American Industrial Hygiene Association.

Clark WW. 1997. Statement of Dr. William Clark, Central Institute for the Deaf. MSHA's Public Hearings: Health Standards for Occupational Noise Exposure in Coal, Metal and Nonmetal Mines. Hearing by the Mine Safety and Health Administration, Washington, DC, May 30. [Online]. Available: http://www.msha.gov/REGS/COMMENTS/NOISE/NOISE.HTM [accessed February 12, 2006].

Cook CK, Hess JE, Tubbs RL. 2001. HETA 2000-0181-2841: Wire Rope Corporation of America, Inc., Sedalia, Missouri. Cincinnati, OH: NIOSH.

Department of the Army. 1998. Medical Services: Hearing Conservation Program. DA PAM 40-501. Washington, DC: Department of the Army.

Dobie RA. 1997. Statement of Dr. Robert Dobie, Chairman, Department of Otolaryngology, University of Texas Health Science Center. In the Matter of: Proposed Rules on Health Standards for Occupational Noise Exposure. Hearing by the Mine Safety and Health Administration, Denver, CO, May 13. [Online]. Available: http://www.msha.gov/REGS/COMMENTS/NOISE/NOISE.HTM [accessed February 12, 2006].

DoD (Department of Defense). 2004. Department of Defense Instruction 6055.12: DoD Hearing Conservation Program. Washington, DC: DoD.

Erway LC, Shiau YW, Davis RR, Krieg E. 1996. Genetics of age-related hearing loss in mice: III. Susceptibility of inbred and F1 hybrid strains to noise-induced hearing loss. *Hearing Research* 93:181–187.

European Parliament and the Council of the European Union. 2003. Directive 2003/10/EC of the European Parliament and of the Council of 6 February 2003 on the minimum health and safety requirements regarding the exposure of workers to the risks arising from physical agents (noise). (Seventeenth individual Directive within the meaning of Article 16(1) of Directive 89/391/EEC). *Official Journal of the European Union* L 042(15/02/2003):38–44.

Franks JR. 1996. Analysis of Audiograms for a Large Cohort of Noise-Exposed Miners. Unpublished technical report. Cincinnati, OH: NIOSH.

Franks JR. 1997a. Initial Results from Analysis of Audiograms for Non-Coal Miners. Cincinnati, OH: NIOSH. Memorandum. June 16.

Franks JR. 1997b. Prevalence of Hearing Loss for Noise-Exposed Metal/Nonmetal Miners. Unpublished technical report. Cincinnati, OH: NIOSH.

Franks JR, Themann CL, Sherris C. 1994. *The NIOSH Compendium of Hearing Protection Devices.* DHHS (NIOSH) Pub. No. 95-105. Cincinnati, OH: NIOSH.

Harney JM, King BF, Tubbs RL, Hayden CS, Kardous CA, Khan A, Mickelsen RL, Wilson RD. 2005. NIOSH Health Hazard Evaluation Report, HETA 2000-0191-2960: Immigration and Naturalization Service, National Firearms Unit, Altoona, Pennsylvania. Cincinnati, OH: NIOSH.

Hayden CS. 2004. Noise control of power tools used in the construction industry—NIOSH/universities partnership case studies. In: Proceedings of NOISE-CON 2004, Baltimore, MD, July 12–14. Pp. 313–317.

Hodgson M, Li D. 2004. Active Control of Workplace Noise Exposure. Final report prepared for the National Institute for Occupational Safety and Health under Grant No. 1 R01 OH003963-01A1. University of British Columbia. October.

ISO (International Organization for Standardization). 1990. ISO 1999. *Acoustics—Determination of Occupational Noise Exposure and Estimation of Noise-Induced Hearing Impairment.* Geneva, Switzerland: ISO.

ISO. 1999. ISO 3741: 1999. *Acoustics—Determination of Sound Power Levels of Noise Sources Using Sound Pressure—Precision Methods for Reverberation Rooms.* Geneva, Switzerland: ISO.

Kardous CH, Franks JR, Davis RR. 2005. NIOSH/NHCA best-practices workshop on impulsive noise. *Noise Control Engineering Journal* 53(2):53–60.

Kovalchik P, Johnson M, Burdisso R, Duda F, Durr M. 2002. A Noise Control for Continuous Miners. Paper for presentation at the 10th International Meeting on Low Frequency Noise and Vibration and Its Control, York, England. September 11–13.

Lick HB. 2001. Ford's annual report to the United Auto Workers (UAW)–Ford National Joint Commission on Health and Safety. In: NIOSH. *Proceedings: Best Practices in Hearing Loss Prevention.* Detroit, Michigan. October 28, 1999. DHHS (NIOSH) Pub. No. 2001-157. Cincinnati, OH: NIOSH. Pp. 9–12.

Lotz WG (NIOSH). 2006a. RE: additional info and document requests. E-mail to L Joellenbeck, Institute of Medicine. January 30.

Lotz WG (NIOSH). 2006b. RE: info request. E-mail to L Joellenbeck, Institute of Medicine. May 26.

Maddux J. 2006. NIOSH Hearing Loss Activities: An OSHA Standards and Guidance Perspective. Presentation to the Committee to Review the NIOSH Hearing Loss Research Program, Meeting II, February 23. Washington, DC.

Matetic RJ. 2006. Research Goal 3: Develop Engineering Controls to Reduce Noise Exposure. Presentation to the Committee to Review the NIOSH Hearing Loss Research Program, Meeting I, January 5. Washington, DC.

McKinney R, Friend RM, Skiles ME. 2004. Program Information Bulletin No. P04-18. Technologically Achievable, Administratively Achievable, and Promising Noise Controls (30 CFR Part 62). Arlington, VA: Mine Safety and Health Administration.

Methner MM, Delaney LJ, and Tubbs RL. 2004. NIOSH Health Hazard Evaluation Report, HETA 2004-0100-2946: Transportation Security Administration, Washington-Dulles International Airport, Dulles, Virginia. Cincinnati, OH: NIOSH.

Michigan State University, Occupational and Environmental Medicine. 2004. Michigan's Project SENSOR (Sentinel Event Notification System for Occupational Risks). East Lansing: Michigan State University. [Online]. Available: http://oem.msu.edu/sensor.asp [accessed January 2006].

MSHA (Mine Safety and Health Administration). 1999. 30 C.F.R. Parts 56, 57, 62, 70, and 71. Health Standards for Occupational Noise Exposure; Final Rule. *Federal Register* 64(176):49548–49634.

Murphy WJ, Franks JR, Krieg EF. 2002. Hearing protector attenuation: Models of attenuation distributions. *Journal of the Acoustical Society of America* 111(5 Part 1):2109–2116.

Murphy WJ, Franks JR, Berger EH, Behar A, Casali JG, Dixon-Ernst C, Krieg EF, Mozo BT, Ohlin DH, Royster JD, Royster LH, Simon SD, Stephenson C. 2004. Development of a new standard laboratory protocol for estimation of the field attenuation of hearing protection devices: Sample size necessary to provide acceptable reproducibility. *Journal of the Acoustical Society of America* 115(1):311–323.

NASA (National Aeronautics and Space Administration). 2006. Hearing Conservation. In: NASA Occupational Health Program Procedures. NPR 1800.1A. Pp. 138–151. [Online]. Available: http://nodis3.gsfc.nasa.gov/displayDir.cfm?Internal_ID=N_PR_1800_001A_&page_name=main [accessed August 2006].

NIDCD (National Institute on Deafness and Other Communication Disorders). 2006. Wise Ears! [Online]. Available: http://www.nidcd.nih.gov/health/wise [accessed May 26, 2006].

NIOSH (National Institute for Occupational Safety and Health). 1978. *Industrial Noise Control Manual*, Rev. ed. Pub. No. 79-117. Cincinnati, OH: NIOSH.

NIOSH. 1980. *Compendium of Materials for Noise Control*. Pub. No. 80-116. Cincinnati, OH: NIOSH.

NIOSH. 1988. A proposed national strategy for the prevention of noise-induced hearing loss. In: *Proposed National Strategies for the Prevention of Leading Work-Related Diseases and Injuries*, Part 2. Cincinnati, OH: NIOSH. Pp. 51–63.

NIOSH. 1996. *Preventing Occupational Hearing Loss—A Practical Guide*. DHHS (NIOSH) Pub. No. 96-110. Cincinnati, OH: NIOSH.

NIOSH. 1998a. *Criteria for a Recommended Standard. Occupational Noise Exposure: Revised Criteria 1998*. DHHS (NIOSH) Pub. No. 98-126. Cincinnati, OH: NIOSH.

NIOSH. 1998b. White Paper: Engineering Noise Controls and Personal Protective Equipment. Paper prepared for Control of Workplace Hazards for the 21st Century: Setting the Research Agenda (conference and workshop), Chicago, March 10–12. [Online]. Available: http://www.cdc.gov/niosh/ctwpnois.html [accessed January 27, 2006].

NIOSH. 2000a. The Hearing Protector Device Compendium. [Online]. Available: http://www.cdc.gov/niosh/topics/noise/hpcomp.html [accessed January 2006].
NIOSH. 2000b. NORA Proposals: NIOSH FY2001 Project Forms. Unpublished document provided to the Committee to Review the NIOSH Hearing Loss Research Program. Cincinnati, OH: NIOSH.
NIOSH. 2001. Identifying Effective Hearing Loss Prevention Strategies (reviewers' comments). Unpublished document provided to the Committee to Review the NIOSH Hearing Loss Research Program. Cincinnati, OH: NIOSH.
NIOSH. 2004. *Worker Health Chartbook, 2004.* DHHS (NIOSH) Pub No. 2004-146. Cincinnati, OH: NIOSH.
NIOSH. 2005a. Collaborations of NIOSH Scientists with Extramural Scientists. Unpublished document provided to the Committee to Review the NIOSH Hearing Loss Research Program. Cincinnati, OH: NIOSH.
NIOSH. 2005b. Databases. In: NIOSH Hearing Loss Research Program: Evidence for the National Academies' Committee to Review the NIOSH Hearing Loss Research Program. Cincinnati, OH: NIOSH. Pp. 8B-1–8B-15.
NIOSH. 2005c. NIOSH FY2006 Project Form. Research Proposal Information Summary: Hearing Loss Prevention for Shipyard Workers. Unpublished document provided to the Committee to Review the NIOSH Hearing Loss Research Program. Cincinnati, OH: NIOSH.
NIOSH. 2005d. NIOSH Hearing Loss Research Program: Overview. In: NIOSH Hearing Loss Research Program: Evidence for the National Academies' Committee to Review the NIOSH Hearing Loss Research Program. Cincinnati, OH: NIOSH. Pp. 19–40.
NIOSH. 2005e. NIOSH Office of Extramural Programs Overview. In: NIOSH Hearing Loss Research Program: Evidence for the National Academies' Committee to Review the NIOSH Hearing Loss Research Program. Cincinnati, OH: NIOSH. Appendix I.
NIOSH. 2005f. Research Goal 1: Contribute to the Development, Implementation, and Evaluation of Effective Hearing Loss Prevention Programs. In: NIOSH Hearing Loss Research Program: Evidence for the National Academies' Committee to Review the NIOSH Hearing Loss Research Program. Cincinnati, OH: NIOSH. Pp. 43–75.
NIOSH. 2005g. Research Goal 2: Reduce Hearing Loss Through Interventions Targeting Personal Protective Equipment. In: NIOSH Hearing Loss Research Program: Evidence for the National Academies' Committee to Review the NIOSH Hearing Loss Research Program. Cincinnati, OH: NIOSH. Pp. 77–99.
NIOSH. 2005h. Research Goal 3: Develop Engineering Controls to Reduce Noise Exposure. In: NIOSH Hearing Loss Research Program: Evidence for the National Academies' Committee to Review the NIOSH Hearing Loss Research Program. Cincinnati, OH: NIOSH. Pp. 101–123.
NIOSH. 2005i. Research Goal 4: Contribute to Reductions in Hearing Loss through the Understanding of Causative Mechanisms. In: NIOSH Hearing Loss Research Program: Evidence for the National Academies' Committee to Review the NIOSH Hearing Loss Research Program. Cincinnati, OH: NIOSH. Pp. 125–155.
NIOSH. 2005j. Partnerships. In: NIOSH Hearing Loss Research Program: Evidence for the National Academies' Committee to Review the NIOSH Hearing Loss Research Program. Cincinnati, OH: NIOSH. Pp. 8C-1–8C-21.
NIOSH. 2005k. Selected NIOSH Sponsored Workshops and Conferences Related to the HLR Program. In: NIOSH Hearing Loss Research Program: Evidence for the National Academies' Committee to Review the NIOSH Hearing Loss Research Program. Cincinnati, OH: NIOSH. Pp. 8A-1–8A-8.

NIOSH. 2006a. Hearing Loss Extramural Award Summary Through FY 2005. Unpublished document provided to the Committee to Review the NIOSH Hearing Loss Research Program. Cincinnati, OH: NIOSH.

NIOSH. 2006b. NIOSH Hearing Loss Research Program: Contracts and CRADAs supported by Intramural Projects. Unpublished document provided to the Committee to Review the NIOSH Hearing Loss Research Program. Cincinnati, OH: NIOSH.

NIOSH. 2006c. NIOSH Hearing Loss Research Program: Funds Received from Other Agencies. Unpublished document provided to the Committee to Review the NIOSH Hearing Loss Research Program. Cincinnati, OH: NIOSH.

NIOSH. 2006d. NIOSH Hearing Loss Research Program: Intramural Projects and Budget Distribution, 1997–2005. Unpublished document provided to the Committee to Review the NIOSH Hearing Loss Research Program. Cincinnati, OH: NIOSH.

NIOSH. 2006e. NIOSH Hearing Loss Research Program: OEP Project Officers (Scientific Program Administrators). Unpublished document provided to the Committee to Review the NIOSH Hearing Loss Research Program. Cincinnati, OH: NIOSH.

NIOSH. 2006f. NIOSH Hearing Loss Research Program: 2005 Futures Workshop. Unpublished document provided to the Committee to Review the NIOSH Hearing Loss Research Program. Cincinnati, OH: NIOSH.

NIOSH. 2006g. NIOSH Program Portfolio. [Online]. Available: http://www.cdc.gov/niosh/programs/ [accessed April 2006].

NIOSH. 2006h. Mining Program Briefing Book. Prepared for the Committee to Review the NIOSH Mining Safety and Health Research Program. Pittsburgh, PA: NIOSH.

OSHA (Occupational Safety and Health Administration). 1999. Appendix IV: D. Hearing Protection Labeling. In: OSHA Technical Manual. [Online]. Available: http://www.osha.gov/dts/osta/otm/noise/hcp/hp_labeling.html [accessed May 4, 2006].

OSHA. 2005. Noise and Hearing Conservation: Controls. [Online]. Available: http://www.osha.gov/SLTC/noisehearingconservation/hazards_solutions.html [accessed May 4, 2006].

Rai A. 2005. Characterization of Noise and Design of Active Noise Control Technology in Longwall Mines. M.S. thesis. West Virginia University, Morgantown, WV.

Rai A, Luo Y, Slagley J, Peng SS, Guffey S. 2005. Survey and Experimental Studies on Engineering Control of Machine Noises in Longwall Mining Faces. Preprint 05-77, SME Annual Meeting, Salt Lake City, UT, February 28–March 2.

Rosenman KD, Panasuk B. 2005. 2004 Annual Report on Work-Related Noise-Induced Hearing Loss in Michigan. Lansing: Michigan State University and Michigan Department of Labor and Economic Growth.

Rotariu M (NIDCD). 2006a. Budget by Program Area for NIDCD. E-mail to K Gilbertson, Institute of Medicine. May 22.

Rotariu M (NIDCD). 2006b. RE: Budget by Program Area for NIDCD. E-mail to K Gilbertson, Institute of Medicine. May 30.

Royster JD, Berger EH, Merry CJ, Nixon CW, Franks JR, Behar A, Casali JG, Dixon-Ernst C, Kieper RW, Mozo BT, Ohlin D, Royster LH. 1996. Development of a new standard laboratory protocol for estimating the field attenuation of hearing protection devices. Part I. Research of Working Group 11, Accredited Standards Committee S12, Noise. *Journal of the Acoustical Society of America* 99:1506–1526.

Royster LH. 1995. In search of a meaningful measure of hearing protector effectiveness. *Spectrum* 12(2):6–13.

Seiler J, Pon M. 2006. MSHA's Perspective on Occupational Noise Exposure Control and Hearing Loss Prevention. Presentation to the Committee to Review the NIOSH Hearing Loss Research Program, Meeting II, February 23. Washington, DC.

Snyder EM, Nemhauser JB. 2003. NIOSH Health Hazard Evaluation Report, HETA 2002-0284-2908: Capitol Heat and Power, Madison, Wisconsin. Cincinnati, OH: NIOSH.

Stephenson M. 2001. Protocol: Hearing Loss Prevention Program for Carpenters. Unpublished document provided to the Committee to Review the NIOSH Hearing Loss Research Program. Cincinnati, OH: NIOSH.

Suter AH. 2002. *Hearing Conservation Manual*, 4th ed. Milwaukee, WI: Council for Accreditation in Occupational Hearing Conservation.

Tubbs RL. 2003. NIOSH Health Hazard Evaluation Report, HETA 2003-0094-2919: Utah Department of Public Safety, Utah Highway Patrol, Salt Lake City, Utah. Cincinnati, OH: NIOSH.

Tubbs RL, Murphy WJ. 2003. NIOSH Health Hazard Evaluation Report, HETA 2002-0131-2898: Fort Collins Police Services, Fort Collins, Colorado. Cincinnati, OH: NIOSH.

USACHPPM (U.S. Army Center for Health Promotion and Preventive Medicine). 2003. Just the Facts: Occupational Ototoxins (Ear Poisons) and Hearing Loss. No. 51-002-0903. Aberdeen Proving Ground, MD: U.S. Army Center for Health Promotion and Preventive Medicine.

U.S. Congress. 1970. The Occupational Safety and Health Act of 1970. Public Law 91-596. Washington, DC: U.S. Congress.

3

Identifying Emerging Issues and Research Areas in Occupational Hearing Loss Prevention

In addition to evaluating the relevance and impact of the work of the National Institute for Occupational Safety and Health (NIOSH) Hearing Loss Research Program to health and safety in the workplace, the committee was charged with assessing the program's targeting of new research areas in occupational safety and health most relevant to future improvements in workplace protection and with identifying emerging issues that appear especially important for NIOSH and the program.

This chapter first provides a brief overview of the Hearing Loss Research Program's process for identifying new or emerging research areas and notes the topics for new research that the program identified in the evidence package (NIOSH, 2005a). The committee's assessment of this process is followed by its suggestions regarding emerging research areas or issues in occupational hearing loss prevention that warrant the consideration of the Hearing Loss Research Program. The committee notes that an in-depth effort to identify new areas of needed research was beyond what was feasible within the time frame and scope of this study. In keeping with the guidance of the Framework Document, the committee has provided suggestions on the basis of the expertise of individual members rather than as the product of a formal process to explore and synthesize recommendations that could be developed through a comprehensive review of the field.

THE HEARING LOSS RESEARCH PROGRAM'S PROCESS FOR IDENTIFYING EMERGING ISSUES AND RESEARCH AREAS IN OCCUPATIONAL HEARING LOSS PREVENTION

In the mid-1990s, the research agenda for the Hearing Loss Research Program emerged primarily from the development of the National Occupational Research Agenda (NORA) and the work done to prepare *Criteria for a Recommended Standard: Occupational Noise Exposure* (NIOSH, 1998a). This chapter focuses on the program's more recent efforts to identify research directions.

As described to the committee, two activities figured prominently in recent efforts by the Hearing Loss Research Program to identify research needs. One of these was a Futures Workshop held in April 2005, and the other was the development of the Mining Research Plan. The Hearing Loss Research Program also responds to input from other sources, including findings in Health Hazard Evaluations (HHEs), the needs of stakeholders in regulatory agencies and elsewhere, and collaborative opportunities that arise in conjunction with the work of other agencies or researchers.

Futures Workshop

The Futures Workshop was planned as a way to develop research goals for the Hearing Loss Research Program for the next 5 to 10 years (NIOSH, 2006a). The meeting included 25 NIOSH staff members, most of whom were from the Hearing Loss Research Program, and 6 outside experts. Participants are listed in Box 3-1. The NIOSH participants included the Hearing Loss Research Program team leaders, who were leading work related to specific research areas, and program audiologists, engineers, and scientists from the Cincinnati and Pittsburgh research laboratories. The committee was informed that as many NIOSH researchers as possible were included to encourage internal discussion of research needs, opportunities, and goals.

The six outside experts gave presentations highlighting important issues in hearing loss research in biology and physiology, epidemiology, instrumentation, control technology, personal protective equipment, and speech communication. The workshop was described as including discussions after each of the presentations and a brainstorming session at the end to generate a list of topics for further consideration by NIOSH hearing loss researchers.

The research needs identified at the Futures Workshop and the discussion that took place at that meeting provided the basis for the section "Emerging Issues" in the evidence package from the Hearing Loss Research Program (NIOSH, 2005a). These topics are listed in Box 3-2.

> **BOX 3-1**
> **Participants in the NIOSH Hearing Loss Prevention Futures Workshop**
> **April 7–8, 2005**
>
> Jim Banach, Vice-President, Quest Technologies
> Elliott Berger, Senior Scientist, E-A-R/Aearo Corporation
> Scott Brueck, NIOSH, Division of Surveillance, Hazard Evaluations, and Field Studies (DSHEFS)
> Adrian Davis, MRC Hearing and Communication Group, School of Education; University of Manchester, United Kingdom
> Rickie Davis, NIOSH, Team Leader, Division of Applied Research and Technology (DART)
> Clayton Doak, NIOSH, Education and Information Division (EID)
> Dennis Driscoll, Noise Control Engineering Consultant, Associates in Acoustics, Inc.
> Scott Earnest, NIOSH, Branch Chief, DART
> John Franks, NIOSH, DART
> Pam Graydon, NIOSH, DART
> Chuck Hayden, NIOSH, DART
> Don Henderson, Professor, State University of New York, Buffalo
> DeLon Hull, NIOSH, Director, Office of Research and Technology Transfer
> David Ingram, NIOSH, Team Leader, Pittsburgh Research Laboratory (PRL)
> Peter Kovalchik, NIOSH, Team Leader, PRL
> Greg Lotz, NIOSH, Associate Director for Science, DART
> R. J. Matetic, NIOSH, Branch Chief, PRL
> Rich McKinley, U.S. Air Force, Wright-Patterson Air Force Base
> Leroy Mickelsen, NIOSH, Deputy Division Director (Acting), DART
> Thais Morata, NIOSH, DART
> Bill Murphy, NIOSH, Team Leader, DART
> Bob Randolph, NIOSH, Team Leader, PRL
> Ray Sinclair, NIOSH, Senior Scientist, Office of the Director
> Carol Stephenson, NIOSH, Branch Chief, EID
> Mark Stephenson, NIOSH, DART
> Christa Themann, NIOSH, DART
> Randy Tubbs, NIOSH, DSHEFS
> Rohit Verma, NIOSH, EID
> Mary Lynn Woebkenberg, NIOSH, Division Director, DART
> Ed Zechmann, NIOSH, DART
>
> SOURCE: NIOSH, 2006a.

**BOX 3-2
Emerging Research Issues Identified by the
Hearing Loss Research Program**

Short Term

Research Goal 1
  Conduct economic cost/benefit analysis of hearing conservation programs and noise controls
Research Goal 2
  Refine fit-check protocol (make as short as possible but still retain accuracy)
Research Goal 3
  Develop basic guidelines on engineering controls and the maintenance of those controls
  Provide leadership to encourage noise education in undergraduate engineering programs
  Publish available noise control solutions (update print and/or web based), with feedback loop
  Develop engineering controls for small businesses

Long Term

Research Goal 1
  Establish a centralized repository of audiometric data that can be accessed by professionals
  Collaborate with partners in education to reach young workers with prevention information and skills
  Strengthen efforts to transfer and disseminate information
Research Goal 3
  Encourage manufacturers to provide noise labels
Research Goal 4
  Establish ongoing surveillance programs for occupational hearing loss and noise exposure
  Repeat large epidemiologic survey of industry (NOES [National Occupational Exposure Survey])
  Collect industry- and job task-specific noise exposure data
  Establish the effectiveness of prophylactic treatments for noise-exposed workers
  Establish recommended exposure limits for mixed exposure of ototoxic chemicals and noise

SOURCE: NIOSH, 2005a, 2006a.

Noted in the evidence package are plans to use the information from the Futures Workshop in developing a strategic plan for the Hearing Loss Research Program. The program is deferring its work on the strategic plan pending completion of the current Institute of Medicine review (Lotz, 2006c).

Mining Research Plan

The Mining Research Plan was developed as part of a strategic planning effort for the NIOSH Mining Safety and Health Research Program, which is undergoing a parallel review by a separate National Academies committee. According to the evidence package for the Mining Safety and Health Research Program review, "the plan was developed to focus the research and prevention activities on the areas of greatest need, as articulated by our customers and stakeholders and illustrated by the surveillance data" (NIOSH, 2006b; also see *http://www.cdc.gov/niosh/nas/mining/whatis-miningresearchplan.htm*). The plan identifies seven strategic goals, each with intermediate goals and performance measures. Strategic Goal 2 is "Reduce noise-induced hearing loss (NIHL) in the mining industry." The intermediate goals and performance measures for Strategic Goal 2 are shown in Box 3-3.

In response to an inquiry from the committee, the Hearing Loss Research Program provided additional information on this portion of the Mining Research Plan. The development of the strategic goal on hearing loss prevention was the responsibility of the Hearing Loss Prevention Branch at the Pittsburgh Research Laboratory. Significant input was provided by important stakeholders through the Noise Partnership Committee, whose members include the United Mine Workers of America, the Bituminous Coal Operators Association, the National Mining Association, and the Mine Safety and Health Administration. These stakeholders contributed surveillance data for consideration in the strategic planning process as well as information on such topics as research barriers to overcome and knowledge gaps related to hearing loss prevention in the mining industry (Lotz, 2006a).

Although the Hearing Loss Research Program noted in the evidence package the existence of the Mining Research Plan and its strategic goal regarding hearing loss prevention, it was not clear how the Mining Research Plan factored into the work and planning of the Hearing Loss Research Program as a whole. Other than in a response to an inquiry from the committee, discussion of the Mining Research Plan or reference to this plan and its performance measures was notably absent from information conveyed to the committee by the Hearing Loss Research Program. The committee believes that the Hearing Loss Research Program could benefit from increased exchange and collaboration among all the program's researchers in the development of research plans and priorities.

> **BOX 3-3**
> **Hearing Loss Prevention Goals in the NIOSH Mining Research Plan**
>
> **Strategic Goal 2:** Reduce noise-induced hearing loss (NIHL) in the mining industry
>
> *Performance Measure:* The shorter-term goal of this research will be achieved if the frequency of noise overexposure of miners is reduced by 25 percent in 5 years and 50 percent in 10 years. However, NIHL usually occurs gradually over a career. The ultimate long-term measure of success is the elimination of new cases of NIHL. The overall success of our hearing loss prevention research will only be seen in 20–30 years.
>
> **Intermediate Goal 2.1:** Develop and maintain a noise source/mine worker exposure database for prioritizing noise control technology.
>
> *Performance Measure:* This goal will be achieved through development of a database of noise source/exposure relationships and equipment noise in all mining commodities and its use by the mining industry and the Mine Safety and Health Administration (MSHA) by 2008.
>
> **Intermediate Goal 2.2:** Develop engineering noise control technologies applicable to surface and underground mining equipment.
>
> *Performance Measure:* The goal for existing noise controls will be achieved by disseminating comprehensive procedures for the evaluation and application of suitable noise controls in underground and surface metal, nonmetal, and coal mines within 3, 4, and 5 years, respectively. The goal for noise control development will be achieved if the industry implements effective new noise controls that reduce the noise overexposures of miners by 25 percent (versus the baseline values) by 2009.
>
> **Intermediate Goal 2.3:** Empower workers to acquire and pursue more effective hearing conservation actions.
>
> *Performance Measure:* This goal will be achieved through measures of dissemination and usage of communication, training, and empowerment tools by 2006. A key measure will be the actual noise dose reduction attained through increased prevention behavior and usage of dose monitoring systems.
>
> **Intermediate Goal 2.4:** Improve the reliability of communication in noisy workplaces.
>
> *Performance Measure:* This goal will be achieved to the extent that key stakeholders acquire, accept, and implement the guidelines on alleviating communications issues by 2006.
>
> SOURCE: NIOSH, 2006b.

Health Hazard Evaluations

HHEs are another potential means for NIOSH to identify research needs. The Health Hazard Evaluation Program is legislatively mandated to provide assistance to employers or employees in evaluating whether chemical, physical, biological, or other agents are hazardous as used or found in the workplace (NIOSH, 1998b). Since the program's inception in 1972, more than 8,000 evaluations have been completed. Of the HHEs completed since 1981, at least 154 have some reference to either hearing loss or noise exposure (see *http://www.cdc.gov/niosh/hhe/*).

One instance in which HHEs helped to identify an area of research for the Hearing Loss Research Program was the observation of widespread hearing loss among 25-year-old carpenters (Bureau of National Affairs, 2001; Tubbs, 2002; Lotz, 2006b). The hearing loss observed in audiograms collected at two conventions of carpenters was worse than might have been anticipated based on the sound levels that had been measured at construction sites and the relatively short work duration based on the workers' ages. The discrepancy between noise level and exposure conditions and observed hearing loss suggested to Hearing Loss Research Program investigators that the impulsive-type noise to which carpenters are exposed may be more damaging than had previously been thought. Following up on these observations, the Hearing Loss Research Program began working with the United Brotherhood of Carpenters to develop a research plan and educational materials to promote awareness of noise hazards and more effective use of hearing protection devices among carpenters, as described in the evidence package for Research Goal 1 (NIOSH, 2005b).

A second example of an HHE leading the Hearing Loss Research Program to more extensive work was an evaluation of impulsive noise exposures undertaken at an indoor firing range belonging to the National Firearms Unit of what was then the U.S. Immigration and Naturalization Service (Harney et al., 2005; Lotz, 2006b). Work carried out for this HHE helped NIOSH identify limitations of existing sound instruments and measurement standards for impulsive noise. The program's research and development efforts to address those limitations are discussed under Research Goal 4 (NIOSH, 2005c).

COMMITTEE ASSESSMENT OF THE HEARING LOSS RESEARCH PROGRAM'S IDENTIFICATION OF EMERGING ISSUES AND RESEARCH AREAS IN OCCUPATIONAL HEARING LOSS PREVENTION

The Framework Document used by the committee to guide its evaluation notes correctly that identifying new or emerging research needs and developing an active research response are among the most challenging aspects of prevention research (see Appendix A). Acknowledging this, as well as the small scale of the program and other challenges noted in Chapter 2, the committee nonetheless has some concerns about the identification of new or emerging research by the Hearing Loss Research Program.

With few exceptions, the list of emerging issues in the evidence package (see Box 3-2) resembles work that the Hearing Loss Research Program described as being under way or among its current research goals. For example, the plans described under "Refine hearing protector fit-testing methods" (NIOSH, 2005a) are difficult to distinguish from efforts described as ongoing in the materials on Research Goal 2. Similarly, "Publish available noise control solutions and updates" reflects ongoing work to update a manual published in 1978, albeit in a way that is web accessible and searchable, with a means for users to contribute additional solutions (NIOSH, 2005a). Although a certain degree of continuity in research effort is necessary and understandable, the committee saw no reference to emerging research topics that reflect areas of research potential over a more distant time horizon or greater imaginative leaps than current projects or their natural follow-ons.

The Framework Document directs the committee to examine the process by which the program identifies new research needs. According to the Hearing Loss Research Program, the Futures Workshop (described above) was the means for generating the list of emerging issues. The evidence package states that the workshop "was convened to develop a strategic research agenda for the HLR program based on input from the scientific and occupational safety and health communities" (NIOSH, 2005d). Supplemental material about the Futures Workshop noted an emphasis on stimulating internal discussion of research needs and opportunities (NIOSH, 2006a).

In the committee's view, the limited reach of the emerging research needs identified by the Hearing Loss Research Program may reflect two problems. One problem is what the committee sees as the limited breadth and diversity of the program's outreach to and input from the communities responsible for occupational hearing loss prevention in the development of the program's research agenda. The other problem is the challenge of setting research priorities while having only minimal data on the occurrence of work-related hearing loss and workers' exposure to noise or ototoxic chemicals, separately or in combination.

The six outside participants in the Futures Workshop are distinguished experts, but they represent a small pool of expertise for the Hearing Loss Research Program to be drawing from in identifying emerging issues. The committee sees a need for much wider outreach to varied research communities for input and ideas to guide the direction of the program's future work. As discussed in Chapter 2 and again in Chapter 4, the program could benefit from expanding the breadth of outside scientific expertise that it draws upon for planning and review of its work. Areas of expertise in which the committee particularly urges the program to seek greater outside contact include noise control engineering and low-noise product design, epidemiology, and management of hearing conservation programs within corporations.

Similarly, targeting research efforts without having adequate current information about the epidemiology of work-related hearing loss is necessarily limiting. Although establishing surveillance programs for occupational hearing loss and noise exposure and conducting a large epidemiologic survey of industry are listed as long-term research topics, these activities need to be made higher priorities in the near term because of the fundamental role that the data they generate should play in the research planning process.

As noted by NIOSH, as well as by the committee elsewhere in this report, the small size of the Hearing Loss Research Program means that the program must necessarily consider its research portfolio carefully. To sustain a leadership role in occupational hearing loss prevention research, however, the Hearing Loss Research Program should actively monitor emerging research needs and opportunities in all aspects of occupational hearing loss prevention. With its limited funding and staffing resources, the program cannot and should not be expected to develop plans to pursue every emerging research area. It should, however, be expected to move into new research areas on the basis of well-informed judgments as to crucial national needs or important concerns that might otherwise be neglected. To address emerging issues effectively, it may well be necessary for the program to gain access to expertise and resources beyond those available within its existing intramural framework. Depending on the subject and the need, appropriate responses may include expanding intramural capacity, targeting extramural funding to work in such areas, collaborating with appropriate stakeholders, or combinations of these. When it addresses such topics through extramural research, the program should expect intramural researchers to actively monitor the outside work and build on the results as appropriate.

EMERGING ISSUES AND RESEARCH AREAS IN OCCUPATIONAL HEARING LOSS PREVENTION IDENTIFIED BY THE EVALUATION COMMITTEE

The committee was asked to include in its report to NIOSH its identification of emerging research needs in occupational hearing loss and noise control. Had this been the central task of the study charge, the committee would have wanted to undertake various activities, which might have included holding a large workshop, or a series of workshops, to draw ideas from many researchers in the several disciplines involved in occupational hearing loss prevention research and to weigh the relative merits of the ideas proposed. Time constraints precluded this approach, and guidance from NIOSH representatives at the initial meeting reinforced the idea that NIOSH would appreciate the results of brainstorming on the part of committee members rather than requiring an in-depth "research needs" assessment.

In this vein, the committee suggests several ideas for consideration. Some of these proposals, like those presented by the Hearing Loss Research Program, are most appropriately characterized as existing research needs that the program should be considering now, whereas others are emerging topics that may deserve increasing attention over the next 10 years. The inclusion of suggestions that describe work similar to activities already being planned by the Hearing Loss Research Program should not be interpreted as implying greater support from the committee for that work than has already been described in Chapter 2.

Near-Term Needs

- Supporting and leading the development of technologies, advocacy, and education related to portable audiometric records (e.g., "smart card technology") for mobile workers. *Rationale:* A growing segment of the workforce, particularly in construction and other underserved industries, experiences frequent changes in employment while continuing to work in high-noise environments.
- Developing robust testing methods and appropriate rating metrics for some of the newer hearing protection device (HPD) technologies, including nonlinear ear plugs, electronic ear plugs, and noise cancellation options at the earplug level. *Rationale:* New HPD technologies are increasingly available and in use; employers and workers need good information on their effectiveness.
- Pursuing research and advocacy related to the development of consensus standards for noise emissions testing of power tools. *Rationale:* Existing standards documents contain insufficient guidance for the conduct of noise emissions testing of power tools for purposes of rating and labeling. Robust and comprehensive testing procedures are a prerequisite to the development of standards for labeling power tools, which will provide guidance for industry "buy-quiet" programs, small business, and the construction sector, as well as the general public.
- Providing leadership in defining occupational hearing loss and exploring improved means of measuring it (e.g., comparing pure-tone averages, otoacoustic emissions, and any other possible approaches; evaluating the appropriateness of "standard threshold shift"). *Rationale:* Averages of hearing levels for pure tones at various sound frequencies have been used for decades to describe hearing loss, but different combinations of frequencies are used for these averages, and newer tech-

nologies such as otoacoustic emissions warrant evaluation in occupational settings. The Hearing Loss Research Program should take the lead in considering ways to measure and define occupational hearing loss.

- Identifying occupations in the modern workplace with high risk of occupational hearing loss from exposure to noise and/or ototoxins. *Rationale:* With the changes in workplace environments and the emergence of new occupations and industries (e.g., in nanotechnology), there is a need to learn whether occupational hearing loss hazards exist in settings beyond those that are a source of long-standing concern and attention.

Longer-Term Needs

- Exploring the interaction between cochlear implants and high sound levels. *Rationale:* Workers with cochlear implants represent a small but growing presence in the workplace. Studies are needed to investigate such issues as the limits of safe sound level exposure for these workers, how workers with cochlear implants should be tested as part of a hearing loss prevention program, and how frequently they should be tested.
- Identifying effective screening methods using new technologies, such as otoacoustic emissions, to improve early identification of high-risk individuals. *Rationale:* Earlier identification of workers who show signs of damage to their hearing may help in ensuring that workers' exposure to noise or ototoxic hazards is being controlled effectively.
- Supporting the development of technologies for hearing-impaired workers that combine amplification and attenuation capabilities for selectable performance. *Rationale:* As the U.S. workforce ages, the number of hearing-impaired workers who need both hearing protection and amplification will increase.
- Developing and promoting standards for product noise emissions labeling. *Rationale:* Work focused on consumer products has been initiated through the Institute of Noise Control Engineering, but the Hearing Loss Research Program could champion a similar effort to advocate for product noise emissions labeling and testing standards for equipment commonly employed in occupational settings.
- Conducting well-designed longitudinal studies of workers exposed and unexposed to occupational noise to determine the long-term effects, if any, of occupational noise exposure after the exposure stops. *Rationale:* Some workers who are exposed to a period of occupational noise are concerned that hearing loss that becomes evident long after such noise exposure ended may be a delayed effect of the earlier exposure. A recent report from the Institute of Medicine (IOM, 2006) found that the available evidence was not sufficient to determine whether perma-

nent noise-induced hearing loss can develop long after the cessation of a given noise exposure.

- Assessing the impact of varied working conditions, such as extended shifts, on occupational hearing loss. *Rationale:* Current noise exposure standards and recommendations are generally based on presumptions of exposure for an 8-hour work day. Current practices in some industry sectors may result in workers routinely being exposed to hearing hazards (i.e., noise, ototoxic chemicals, or both) during longer work days of 12 hours or more.

CONCLUSION

Identification of emerging concerns is an important and challenging aspect of the Hearing Loss Research Program's stated mission "to provide national and world leadership to reduce the prevalence of occupational hearing loss through a focused program of research and prevention." The committee noted room for improvement in the program's recent approach to this task. Although the committee suggested additional areas for consideration, it emphasizes that this important task warrants more extensive expert input and evaluation than the committee could provide in the context of its review. Whether or not the NIOSH Hearing Loss Research Program is able to undertake activities proposed by the committee, the program should aim to be at the forefront of efforts to review and define needs in occupational hearing loss prevention and to promote opportunities to pursue new and innovative to ways to respond to those needs.

REFERENCES

Bureau of National Affairs. 2001. Hearing loss expected by carpenters, but study finds workers fear tinnitus more. *Occupational Safety and Health Reporter* 31(April 5): 303–305. [Online]. Available: http://www.cdc.gov/elcosh/docs/d0400/d000452/d000452.html [accessed May 9, 2006].

Harney JM, King BF, Tubbs RL, Hayden CS, Kardous CA, Khan A, Mickelsen RL, Wilson RD. 2005. NIOSH Health Hazard Evaluation Report, HETA 2000-0191-2960: Immigration and Naturalization Service, National Firearms Unit, Altoona, Pennsylvania. Cincinnati, OH: NIOSH.

IOM (Institute of Medicine). 2006. *Noise and Military Service: Implications for Hearing Loss and Tinnitus.* Humes LE, Joellenbeck LM, Durch JS, eds. Washington, DC: The National Academies Press.

Lotz WG (NIOSH). 2006a. RE: additional info and document requests. E-mail to L Joellenbeck, Institute of Medicine. January 30.

Lotz WG (NIOSH). 2006b. RE: info request. E-mail to L Joellenbeck, Institute of Medicine. May 26.

Lotz WG (NIOSH). 2006c. Re: update on timing, and question. E-mail to L Joellenbeck, Institute of Medicine. June 14.

NIOSH (National Institute for Occupational Safety and Health). 1998a. *Criteria for a Recommended Standard. Occupational Noise Exposure: Revised Criteria 1998*. DHHS (NIOSH) Pub. No. 98-126. Cincinnati, OH: NIOSH.

NIOSH. 1998b. *Health Hazard Evaluations: Noise and Hearing Loss 1986–1997*. DHHS (NIOSH) Pub. No. 99-106. Cincinnati, OH: NIOSH.

NIOSH. 2005a. Emerging Issues. In: NIOSH Hearing Loss Research Program: Evidence for the National Academies' Committee to Review the NIOSH Hearing Loss Research Program. Cincinnati, OH: NIOSH. Pp. 157–162.

NIOSH. 2005b. Research Goal 1: Contribute to the Development, Implementation, and Evaluation of Effective Hearing Loss Prevention Programs. In: NIOSH Hearing Loss Research Program: Evidence for the National Academies' Committee to Review the NIOSH Hearing Loss Research Program. Cincinnati, OH: NIOSH. Pp. 43–75.

NIOSH. 2005c. Research Goal 4: Contribute to Reductions in Hearing Loss through the Understanding of Causative Mechanisms. In: NIOSH Hearing Loss Research Program: Evidence for the National Academies' Committee to Review the NIOSH Hearing Loss Research Program. Cincinnati, OH: NIOSH. Pp. 125–155.

NIOSH. 2005d. Selected NIOSH Sponsored Workshops and Conferences Related to the HLR Program. In: NIOSH Hearing Loss Research Program: Evidence for the National Academies' Committee to Review the NIOSH Hearing Loss Research Program. Cincinnati, OH: NIOSH. Pp. 8A-1–8A-8.

NIOSH. 2006a. NIOSH Hearing Loss Research Program: 2005 Futures Workshop. Unpublished document provided to the Committee to Review the NIOSH Hearing Loss Research Program. Cincinnati, OH: NIOSH.

NIOSH. 2006b. 1.5 Mining Research Plan (Strategic Goals). In: NIOSH Mining Program Briefing Book. Unpublished document prepared for the Committee to Review the NIOSH Mining Safety and Health Research Program. Pittsburgh, PA: NIOSH. Pp. 33–53.

Tubbs RL. 2002. Memorandum: Close-out of HETA 95-0249; HETA 96-0007. Unpublished document provided to the Committee to Review the NIOSH Hearing Loss Research Program. Cincinnati, OH: NIOSH.

4

Recommendations for Program Improvement

As the only federal research program focused specifically on the challenge of preventing occupational hearing loss, the Hearing Loss Research Program within the National Institute for Occupational Safety and Health (NIOSH) should be an undisputed leader and source of expertise in the fields of occupational hearing loss research, including hearing loss prevention programs, hearing protection, noise control engineering for occupational hearing loss prevention, and occupational hearing loss surveillance and risk factors. From its evaluation of the relevance and impact of this NIOSH program (Chapter 2) and its assessment of the identification of new research areas (Chapter 3), the Committee to Review the NIOSH Hearing Loss Research Program identified several potential opportunities to improve the relevance of the program's work and strengthen its impact on reducing occupational hearing loss. This chapter provides the committee's recommendations for improvement of the Hearing Loss Research Program. The committee recognizes that some of these recommendations carry resource implications that have not been fully explored here. It hopes that NIOSH will place a high enough value on the Hearing Loss Research Program to give serious consideration to finding ways to respond to these opportunities for improvement.

PROGRAM MANAGEMENT IN A MATRIX ENVIRONMENT

The NIOSH Hearing Loss Research Program operates in a matrix environment, as do many other NIOSH research programs. This approach to program management offers benefits to the organization as a whole, but it poses challenges for the Hearing Loss Research Program's ability to develop and implement a program plan and to allocate resources among the varied research needs related to occupational hearing loss prevention. The committee notes that even the most talented leadership will find it difficult to successfully manage a program distributed across separate organizational units and to catalyze the planning and mobilization of resources necessary for a cohesive program. The small size of the program also demands skill in setting priorities for program activities and allocation of program resources. The program as a whole requires leadership specifically dedicated to championing a better Hearing Loss Research Program, as do each of the program areas represented by the four research goals.

In addition to having excellent management skills, leaders should be well-regarded experts in hearing loss prevention, noise control engineering, or surveillance methods. They should be involved with other organizations through activities such as participation in standards committees, advisory panels, and boards. The program's leaders should also bring experience in implementing hearing loss prevention or noise control engineering practices in the field.

Since 1996, the Hearing Loss Research Program has had to respond to significant organizational and leadership challenges. The incorporation of activities at the Pittsburgh Research Laboratory added a new and physically separated component to the program. The Hearing Loss Research Program also lost two experienced and recognized leaders in the field. Furthermore, the Hearing Loss Research Program has had to respond to the NIOSH-wide effort to look toward a second decade of the National Occupational Research Agenda (NORA) and the demands of preparing for the review by this committee.

Although the Hearing Loss Research Program has persevered admirably during these transitional times, the committee sees a need to foster leadership that can provide coherence to the program, increase collaboration, and serve as an effective advocate within the matrix environment in which it operates. The committee is encouraged to see that NIOSH has recently appointed from within the NIOSH management staff an overall program manager who is expected to monitor the program's activities and resources. In this role, the program manager will have an advisory and consultative relationship with the organizational units in which the Hearing Loss Research Program's work is done, but he will not have authority to mandate the allocation of resources to the program as a whole or its components. The program manager did not make a formal presentation to the committee, and even though he is new to this position, it would have been valuable to the committee to hear his views on the program and the Institute of Medicine review.

1. **Foster effective leadership.** NIOSH should ensure that the Hearing Loss Research Program and its components have leadership with appropriate technical expertise as well as skills in managing in a complex environment, mobilizing resources, promoting collaboration within the program, and increasing program coherence. All of these leaders must serve as champions of the program within and outside NIOSH and help to garner adequate resources and recruit expertise. The leaders should be respected and involved in the hearing loss prevention community and in their own fields of expertise. NIOSH should provide the overall program leader with sufficient authority to make appropriate program and budgetary decisions.

It bears repeating that the leaders of the Hearing Loss Research Program must contend with a small budget—about $7.5 million in fiscal year (FY) 2005—much of which is reserved for work related to mining or for extramural research. The committee urges NIOSH to consider the need for program resources that are commensurate with a more robust pursuit of the program's goals and with sustaining the continuity of the most relevant research in specific program areas.

ACCESS TO INTRAMURAL AND EXTRAMURAL EXPERTISE

As described in Chapters 2 and 3, the committee is concerned that the Hearing Loss Research Program has lacked adequate internal technical expertise, especially in the specialized areas of epidemiology and noise control engineering, and has appeared to rely on a fairly narrow group of external experts for input and collaboration. For the program to hold the position of national leadership in occupational hearing loss prevention and noise control research, it must draw on outstanding members of the communities responsible for the prevention of occupational hearing loss (as detailed in Chapter 1) both within and outside the program.

The committee commends the efforts by the management of the Hearing Loss Research Program to increase capabilities of its staff by supporting graduate education in fields such as noise control engineering. Although this approach can supplement the program's resources, it is not a substitute for the recruitment of senior-level researchers with demonstrated expertise in areas essential to the effective performance of the program. Similarly, seeking contributions to program planning discussions from outside experts is appropriate, but relying on a small set of contributors (e.g., only six outside participants at the Futures Workshop) does not provide sufficient breadth and depth of expertise.

As the Hearing Loss Research Program garners additional internal expertise, it should also broaden and strengthen its ties to sources of external scientific, hearing loss prevention, and noise control engineering expertise, such as other federal agencies, industry, and the military. With additional expertise, the program will be better positioned to have an impact on occupational hearing loss through its current portfolio as well as to move into emerging research areas for the future.

2. **Recruit additional expert researchers to the NIOSH Hearing Loss Research Program staff.** The Hearing Loss Research Program should recruit and retain experienced professionals with recognized expertise in the fields of epidemiology and noise control engineering who can exercise leadership in planning, conducting, and evaluating the program's work in these crucial areas. It is essential for the program to make gaining this additional expertise a priority.
3. **Expand access to outside expertise.** The program should make efforts to draw upon a wider representation of the communities responsible for the prevention of occupational hearing loss as reviewers, conference participants, and collaborators. As part of this effort, the program should strengthen ties to the National Institute on Deafness and Other Communication Disorders and other components of the National Institutes of Health to benefit from additional interactions with the scientific researchers there. The program should also explore collaborations with noise control engineers inside and outside the federal government.

PROGRAM PLANNING

Even as the National Academies' evaluation of up to 15 different NIOSH research programs is under way, NIOSH as a whole is undergoing changes. NIOSH has organized its program portfolio into 8 NORA programs representing industrial sectors, 15 cross-sector programs organized around adverse health outcomes (such as hearing loss), and 7 coordinated emphasis areas (*http://www.cdc.gov/niosh/programs/*) (NIOSH, 2006). It is developing strategic plans for each of its research programs, and new emphasis is being placed on the translation and application of scientific knowledge to the workplace with the assistance of the NIOSH Office of Research and Technology Transfer. The committee commends NIOSH for its continued striving for improvement as an organization.

The Hearing Loss Research Program has acknowledged that until recently it has managed more by opportunity than by objective. Although it may not be feasible for such a small program to manage entirely by objective, and the group has proven itself adept at leveraging opportunities, the committee urges additional efforts to focus its limited resources on its most relevant goals, as discussed in Chapter 2.

An important input to this planning can be the research needs of the Occupational Safety and Health Administration (OSHA) and the Mine Safety and Health Administration (MSHA). It appears to the committee that the mechanisms through which the Hearing Loss Research Program anticipates the early research needs of its regulatory partners are not sufficiently consistent and systematic. Although technical staffs at NIOSH, OSHA, and MSHA appear to work well together, there does not seem to be an effective joint planning process for regulatory activities. This is not entirely within NIOSH's control, but it deserves greater attention in the future.

4. **Develop a strategic plan.** The Hearing Loss Research Program should develop a strategic plan that takes into account the strengths, weaknesses, and external factors identified in this evaluation. It should reflect a focus on the program's mission and serve to guide decision making about the value of projects and proposed collaborations. It should also reflect coordination with the strategic plans developed by the sector-based NIOSH research programs that may need to address hearing loss as one of several health hazards faced by the workforce.

5. **Use surveillance data as well as stakeholder input to identify priorities.** The Hearing Loss Research Program should make the rationale for its research prioritization more explicit, using analyses of surveillance data to the extent possible as well as the concerns and interests of stakeholders from a variety of industrial sectors to guide allocations of resources and effort.

6. **Use information from evaluation of hearing loss prevention measures to guide program planning.** The Hearing Loss Research Program should use information gained from evaluation of the effectiveness of its program activities to help identify approaches to hearing loss prevention that should be emphasized, revised, or possibly discontinued.

7. **Systematize collaboration with regulatory partners.** The Hearing Loss Research Program should establish regular means for conferring with OSHA, MSHA, and the Environmental Protection Agency to better anticipate research needs relevant to regulatory decision making.

EVALUATION OF HEARING LOSS PREVENTION MEASURES

Developing and disseminating "best practices" and training methods for hearing loss prevention programs to apply scientific understanding to the workplace has been an important contribution of the Hearing Loss Research Program and is the focus of Research Goal 1. In its evidence package, the program notes the need for intervention effectiveness research designed to validate best practices for each of the seven components of hearing loss prevention programs advocated by NIOSH (2005). The committee underscores the importance of evaluation of the effectiveness of all program activities, including the dissemination of the educational material that the program develops, as a crucial step in ensuring that the Hearing Loss Research Program serves as a leader in producing evidence-based guidance on hearing loss prevention.

8. **Place greater emphasis on evaluation of the effectiveness of hearing loss prevention measures on the basis of outcomes that are as closely related as possible to reducing noise exposure and the incidence of occupational hearing loss.** The Hearing Loss Research Program should implement consistent and concerted evaluation activities that inform and focus its work on hearing loss prevention. Prospective evaluations of the recommended components of hearing loss prevention programs are needed to determine which features have the most significant impacts on reducing noise exposure levels or hearing loss incidence rates. These evaluations should address actual (not just intended) worker and employer behavior and the end results of exposure levels and hearing loss.

SURVEILLANCE ACTIVITIES

The Hearing Loss Research Program notes in its evidence package that the lack of surveillance data on workers' noise exposures and the incidence and severity of occupational hearing loss is one of the fundamental knowledge gaps in the field. The committee agrees and underscores the importance of surveillance data and their careful analysis to help guide priority setting for research in occupational health and safety and for evaluation of program activities. Although the Hearing Loss Research Program has participated in several different efforts (described in Chapter 2) to address the lack of surveillance data, the current program approaches are piecemeal and require expansion of their conceptual framework and measurement methods. To maintain an appropriate scientific leadership role in the field of occupational hearing loss prevention, the Hearing Loss Research Program needs to increase its emphasis on and expertise in surveillance. Doing so will require resources commensurate with the task. It will also require the leadership of one or more experienced epidemiologists integrated into the program staff (see Recommendation 2 above). Relying on ad hoc epidemiologic assistance is not sufficient.

With additional program epidemiology and surveillance expertise, the Hearing Loss Research Program should plan means to gather and analyze new data on the occurrence of hearing loss and hazardous noise exposure. Possible and complementary approaches, as outlined in a recent National Academies report on health and safety needs of older workers (NRC and IOM, 2004), include initiating new longitudinal studies, increasing information gathered from ongoing longitudinal surveys (as the Hearing Loss Research Program has done in working with OSHA), collaborating with the Bureau of Labor Statistics for a comprehensive review of occupational injury or illness reporting systems, and developing a database to characterize levels of exposures associated with work (as the program has been doing for mining).

9. **Initiate national surveillance for occupational hearing loss and hazardous noise.** The Hearing Loss Research Program should rally expertise and resources to lead surveillance of the incidence and prevalence of work-related hearing loss and the occurrence of exposure to hazardous noise levels in occupational settings in the United States. Surveillance efforts should be accompanied by plans for appropriate analyses of the data.

NOISE CONTROL PERSPECTIVE

Following the industrial hygiene tradition of the "hierarchy of controls," noise control engineering should be the primary approach to the prevention of hearing loss. In reality, employers frequently turn first to administrative controls or hearing protection devices to decrease workers' exposure to hazardous noise. Perhaps as a result, the research emphasis within the Hearing Loss Research Program has also been on aspects of hearing loss prevention other than noise control. Over the past decade, substantially more of the program's resources have been brought to bear on noise control engineering, but those resources have been directed primarily to the mining industry. Although congressional guidance has resulted in most of this funding being devoted to a single industrial sector, the committee sees it as the mission of the Hearing Loss Research Program to pursue broader applications of its work on noise control engineering. To help identify the potential for broader applications of mining-related work, the committee urges increased collaboration between the Pittsburgh- and Cincinnati-based researchers.

10. **Integrate the noise control engineering perspective into overall program efforts for all sectors.** The Hearing Loss Research Program should apply its dissemination expertise to further emphasize the application of "quiet by design," "buy quiet," and engineered noise control approaches to industrial settings as part of hearing loss prevention programs.
11. **Develop noise control engineering approaches for non-mining sectors.** The Hearing Loss Research Program should increase efforts to develop noise control approaches applicable in industrial sectors outside mining where workers are also at risk from hazardous noise. Where possible, "dual-use" applications from work done in mining could help bring noise reduction benefit to both miners and workers from other industrial sectors.
12. **Increase the visibility of noise control engineering as a component of the Hearing Loss Research Program.** The Hearing Loss Research Program should use means such as periodic workshops on noise control engineering topics to raise the visibility of its noise control engineering projects within the field. Such workshops can facilitate information exchange, can provide specialized technical training, and may attract qualified professionals who can serve as advisers, consultants, collaborators, or recruits to the NIOSH program.
13. **Accredit laboratories used to conduct studies for the Hearing Loss Research Program.** The Hearing Loss Research Program should work to achieve accreditation of all laboratories that are involved in the acquisition of data that are published or shared externally. To the extent possible, testing on behalf of the NIOSH intramural program should be carried out at facilities owned or controlled by NIOSH.

EXTRAMURAL RESEARCH

Slightly more than $14 million, or about 30 percent of the total expenditures of the NIOSH Hearing Loss Research Program between FY 1997 and FY 2005, was directed toward extramural, competitive application projects related to hearing loss or noise control engineering. With the exception of one Request for Application (RFA) in 2001, the Hearing Loss Research Program has relied on the investigator-initiated pipeline for extramural research projects rather than issuing requests for targeted extramural proposals. The extramural research that has resulted includes important contributions to the knowledge base in this field and has facilitated some productive collaborations with Hearing Loss Research Program researchers. In some cases, however, intramural researchers have not made themselves aware of relevant extramural research, which may have resulted in limited opportunities for effective collaboration.

The committee notes the potential for greater use of RFAs and focused Program Announcements (PAs) to direct some extramural funding toward high-priority research topics that complement the program's intramural work. The Hearing Loss Research Program may also want to further pursue efforts to invite outside researchers to work at NIOSH facilities on a temporary basis and at little cost to the program. The committee recommends the following steps to maximize the benefit that the extramural funding might bring to realizing the mission of the Hearing Loss Research Program.

14. **Target more of the extramural research funding.** The Hearing Loss Research Program should increase its use of Requests for Applications and focused Program Announcements to target more of its extramural research funding toward program priority areas.
15. **Increase collaboration and mutual awareness of ongoing work among intramural and extramural researchers.** For the Hearing Loss Research Program to maximize the benefit of extramural research, it is important for intramural and extramural researchers to each be aware of the work that the others are doing relevant to occupational hearing loss or noise control. Where appropriate, intramural researchers should be building upon extramural work within the Hearing Loss Research Program. Toward this end, after a grant has been awarded, NIOSH should facilitate increased communication between intra- and extramural researchers.

REFERENCES

NIOSH (National Institute for Occupational Safety and Health). 2005. Research Goal 1: Contribute to the Development, Implementation, and Evaluation of Effective Hearing Loss Prevention Programs. In: NIOSH Hearing Loss Research Program: Evidence for the National Academies' Committee to Review the NIOSH Hearing Loss Research Program. Cincinnati, OH: NIOSH. Pp. 43–75.

NIOSH. 2006. NIOSH Program Portfolio. [Online]. Available: http://www.cdc.gov/niosh/programs/ [accessed April 2006].

NRC and IOM (National Research Council and Institute of Medicine). 2004. *Health and Safety Needs of Older Workers.* Wegman DH, McGee JP, eds. Washington, DC: The National Academies Press.

A

Framework for the Review of Research Programs of the National Institute for Occupational Safety and Health*

This is a document prepared by the National Academies' Committee for the Review of NIOSH Research Programs,[1] also referred to as the Framework Committee. This document is not a formal report of the National Academies—rather, it is a framework proposed for use by a number of National Academies committees that will be reviewing research in various research programs and health-outcomes programs. This version will be posted on the website of the National Academies and NIOSH for review. It is a working document that will be subject to change by the Framework Committee aimed at improving its

---

*Version of 12/19/05.

[1] Members of the National Academies' Committee for the Review of NIOSH Research Programs include: David Wegman (Chair; University of Massachusetts Lowell School of Health and Environment), William Bunn, III (International Truck and Engine Corporation), Carlos Camargo (Harvard Medical School), Letitia Davis (Massachusetts Department of Public Health), James Dearing (Ohio University), Fred Mettler, Jr. (University of New Mexico School of Medicine), Franklin Mirer (United Automobile, Aerospace, and Agricultural Implement Workers of America), Jacqueline Nowell (United Food and Commercial Workers International Union), Raja Ramani (Pennsylvania State University), Jorma Rantanen (Finnish Institute of Occupational Health), Rosemary Sokas (University of Illinois at Chicago School of Public Health), Richard Tucker (Tucker and Tucker Consultants, Inc., and University of Texas at Austin), Joseph Wholey (University of Southern California School of Policy, Planning, and Development), and James Zuiches (Washington State University).

relevance on the basis of responses received from evaluation committee members, NIOSH, stakeholders, and the general public before and during the course of the assessments conducted by independent evaluation committees of up to 15 research programs and health-outcomes programs.

All public comments submitted to the Committee for the Review of NIOSH Research Programs will be included in the Public Access File for this study as provided in the National Academies Terms of Use (www.nationalacademies.org/legal/terms.html). Please keep in mind that if you directly disclose personal information in your written comments, this information may be collected and used by others.

For inquiries related to this document, or for the most current document version, please contact Evan Douple (edouple@nas.edu) or Sammantha Magsino (smagsino@nas.edu) of the National Academies.

APPENDIX A

CONTENTS

Acronyms
I. Overview of Charge
    I.A. NIOSH Strategic Goals and Operational Plan
    I.B. Information from Other Evaluations
    I.C. Evaluation Committees
    I.D. Evaluation Committees' Information Needs
II. Summary of Evaluation Process
    II.A. The Evaluation Flow Chart (Figure 2)
    II.B. Steps in Program Evaluation
    II.C. Assessing Relevance
    II.D. Assessing Impact
III. Evaluation of NIOSH Research Programs—the Process
    III.A. Analysis of External Factors Relevant to the NIOSH Program
        III.A.1. Overview
        III.A.2. Considerations for Discussion
    III.B. Evaluating NIOSH Research Programs (Addressing Charges 1 and 2)
        III.B.1. Identifying Period of Time to be Evaluated
        III.B.2. Identification of Major Challenges (Circle in Figure 2)
        III.B.3. Analysis of NIOSH Program Strategic Goals and Objectives (Box A in Figure 2)
        III.B.4. Review of Inputs (Box B in Figure 2)
        III.B.5. Review of Activities (Box C in Figure 2)
        III.B.6. Review of Outputs (Box D in Figure 2)
        III.B.7. Review of Intermediate Outcomes (Box E in Figure 2)
        III.B.8. Review of End Outcomes (Box F in Figure 2)
        III.B.9. Review of Other Outcomes
        III.B.10. Summary Evaluation Ratings and Rationale
    III.C. Identifying Significant Emerging Research (Addressing Charge 3)
IV. Evaluation Committee Report Template
V. Framework Committee Final Report

Figure 1   The NIOSH operational plan presented as a logic model
Figure 2   Flow chart for the evaluation of the NIOSH research program

Table 1   NORA High-priority Research Areas by Category
Table 2   Examples of NIOSH Program Research and Transfer Activities
Table 3   Examples of a Variety of Scientific Information Outputs
Table 4   Evaluation Committee Worksheet to Assess Research Programs and Subprograms

ACRONYMS

ABLES	Adult Blood Lead Epidemiology and Surveillance
ACOEM	American College of Occupational and Environmental Medicine
AOEC	Association of Occupational and Environmental Clinics
BLS	Bureau of Labor Statistics
CDC	Centers for Disease Control and Prevention
EC	Evaluation Committee
FACE	Fatality Assessment Control and Evaluation
FC	Framework Committee
HHE	Health Hazard Evaluations
MSHA	Mine Safety and Health Administration
NEISS	National Electronic Injury Surveillance System
NIOSH	National Institute for Occupational Safety and Health
NORA	National Occupational Research Agenda
NORA1	National Occupational Research Agenda 1996-2005
NORA2	National Occupational Research Agenda 2005-Forward
OSHA	Occupational Safety and Health Administration
OSHAct	Occupational Safety and Health Act of 1970
OSH Review Commission	Occupational Safety and Health Review Commission
PART	Performance Assessment Rating Tool
PEL	Permissible Exposure Limits
SENSOR	Sentinel Event Notification System of Occupational Risks
TMT	Tools, Methods, or Technologies

APPENDIX A

In September 2004, the National Institute for Occupational Safety and Health (NIOSH) contracted with the National Academies to conduct a review of NIOSH research programs. The goal of this multiphase effort is to assist NIOSH in increasing the impact of its research efforts in reducing workplace illnesses and injuries and improving occupational safety and health. The National Academies agreed to conduct this review and assigned the task to the Division on Earth and Life Studies and the Institute of Medicine.

The National Academies appointed a committee of 14 members, including persons with expertise in occupational medicine and health, industrial health and safety, industrial hygiene, epidemiology, civil and mining engineering, sociology, program evaluation, communication, and toxicology; representatives of industry and of the workforce; and a scientist experienced in international occupational-health issues. The Committee on the Review of NIOSH Research Programs, referred to as the Framework Committee (FC), held meetings during 2005 on May 5-6 and July 7-8 in Washington, DC, and on August 15-16 in Woods Hole and Falmouth, MA.

This document is not a report of the National Academies; rather, it presents the evaluation framework developed by the FC to serve as a guideline and structure for NIOSH program reviews by Evaluation Committees (ECs) to be appointed by various divisions and boards of the National Academies. The ECs will use this framework in reviewing as many as 15 NIOSH research programs during a 5-year period. This is a working document. It is shared with NIOSH and the public. The framework and criteria may be modified by the FC on the basis of responses it receives from the ECs and other sources. It is incumbent upon the ECs to consult with the FC if portions of the evaluation framework presented here are inappropriate for the specific program under review.

I. OVERVIEW OF CHARGE

At the first meeting of the FC, Lewis Wade, NIOSH senior science advisor, emphasized that the reviews should focus on evaluating NIOSH's research programs impact and relevance to health and safety in the workplace. In developing a framework, the FC was asked to address the following:

1. Evaluation committee assessment of progress in reducing workplace illnesses and injuries facilitated by occupational safety and health research through (a) an analysis of relevant data about workplace illnesses and injuries for the program activity, and (b) an evaluation of the effect that NIOSH research has had in reducing illnesses and injuries. The evaluation committees will rate the performance of each program for impact of the

program in the workplace. Impact may be assessed directly or, as necessary, using intermediate outcomes to estimate impact. Qualitative narrative evaluations may also be appropriate under certain circumstances.
2. Evaluation committee assessment of progress in targeting new research to the areas of occupational safety and health most relevant to future improvements in workplace protection.
3. Evaluation committee identification of significant emerging research areas which appear especially important in terms of their relevance to the mission of NIOSH.

Those three charges constitute the scope of work of the individually appointed, independent ECs formed by the National Academies.

I.A. NIOSH Strategic Goals and Operational Plan

As a prelude to understanding the NIOSH strategic goals and operational plan, NIOSH research efforts should be understood in the context of the Occupational Safety and Health Act (OSHAct) under which it was created. The OSHAct identifies workplace safety and health to be a national priority and gives employers the responsibility for controlling hazards and preventing workplace injury and illness. The act creates an organizational framework for doing this, with complementary roles and responsibilities assigned to employers and employees, OSHA, the States, the OSH Review Commission, and NIOSH. As one component of a national strategy the act recognizes NIOSH's roles and responsibilities to be supportive and indirect—NIOSH's research, training programs, criteria and recommendations are all intended to be used to inform and assist those actually responsible for hazard control (OSHAct Section 2b and Sections 20 and 22).

Section 2b of the OSHAct describes thirteen interdependent means of accomplishing the national goal, one of which is "by providing for research . . . and by developing innovative methods . . . for dealing with occupational safety and health problems." Sections 20 and 22 give the responsibility for this research to NIOSH. In addition, NIOSH is given related responsibilities including: the development of criteria to guide prevention of work-related injury or illness, development of regulations reporting on the employee exposures to harmful agents, the establishment of medical examinations programs or tests to determine illness incidence and susceptibility, publication of a list of all known toxic substances, the assessment of potentially toxic effects or risk associated with workplace exposures in specific settings, the conduct of education programs for relevant professionals to carry out the OSHAct purposes, and assisting the Secretary of Labor regarding education programs for employees and employers in hazard recognition and control.

The NIOSH mission is "to provide national and world leadership to prevent work-related illness, injury, disability, and death by gathering information, conducting scientific research, and translating the knowledge gained into products and services". To fulfill its mission, NIOSH has established the following strategic goals:[2]

- **Goal 1: Conduct research to reduce work-related illnesses and injuries.**
  - Track work-related hazards, exposures, illnesses, and injuries for prevention.
  - Generate new knowledge through intramural and extramural research programs.
  - Develop innovative solutions for difficult-to-solve problems in high-risk industrial sectors.
- **Goal 2: Promote safe and healthy workplaces through interventions, recommendations, and capacity-building.**
  - Enhance the relevance and utility of recommendations and guidance.
  - Transfer research findings, technologies, and information into practice.
  - Build capacity to address traditional and emerging hazards.
- **Goal 3: Enhance global workplace safety and health through international collaborations.**
  - Take a leadership role in developing a global network of occupational health centers.
  - Investigate alternative approaches to workplace illness and injury reduction and provide technical assistance to put solutions in place.
  - Build global professional capacity to address workplace hazards through training, information sharing, and research experience.

In 1994, NIOSH embarked on a national partnership effort to identify research priorities to guide occupational health and safety research for the next decade. The National Occupational Research Agenda (NORA) identified 21 high-priority research areas (see Table 1). NORA was intended not only for NIOSH but for the entire occupational health community. Approaching the 10-year anniversary of NORA, NIOSH is working with its partners to update the research agenda. In the second decade of NORA, an approach based on industry sectors will be pursued. NIOSH and its partners will form sector research councils that will work

---

[2] See also http://www.cdc.gov/niosh/docs/strategic/.

TABLE 1 NORA High-Priority Research Areas by Category

Category	Priority Research Area
Disease and injury	Allergic and irritant dermatitis
	Asthma and chronic obstructive pulmonary disease
	Fertility and pregnancy abnormalities
	Hearing loss
	Infectious diseases
	Low-back disorders
	Musculoskeletal disorders of upper extremities
	Trauma
Work environment and workforce	Emerging technologies
	Indoor environment
	Mixed exposures
	Organization of work
	Special populations at risk
Research tools and approaches	Cancer research methods
	Control technology and personal protective equipment
	Exposure-assessment methods
	Health-services research
	Intervention-effectiveness research
	Risk-assessment methods
	Social and economic consequences of workplace illness and injury
	Surveillance research methods

to establish sector-specific research goals and objectives. Emphasis will be placed on moving research to practice in workplaces through sector-based partnerships.

Figure 1 is the NIOSH operational plan presented as a logic model[3] of the path from inputs to outcomes for each NIOSH research program. The FC adapted the model to develop its framework. NIOSH will provide similar logic models relevant to each research program evaluated by an EC.

I.B. Information from Other Evaluations

The FC is aware that several NIOSH programs have already been subjected to evaluation by internal and external bodies. Those evaluations range from overall assessments of NIOSH, such as the recent 2005 Performance Assessment Rating

---

[3] Developed by NIOSH with the assistance of the RAND Corporation.

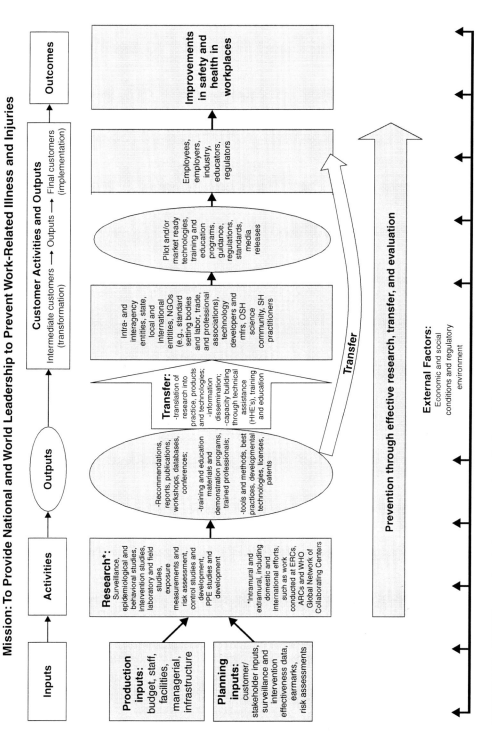

FIGURE 1 The NIOSH operational plan presented as a logic model.

Tool (PART) review,[4] to evaluation of research program elements such as any external scientific program reviews. The ECs should review all available prior reviews. Although it is important to consider all prior reviews in the present evaluation to aid in understanding the evolution of the programs and program elements, the ECs' evaluations of NIOSH's programs are independent of the prior reviews and evaluations.

I.C. Evaluation Committees

Individual ECs will be formed through a process consistent with the rules of the National Academies for the formation of balanced committees. The committees will be composed of persons with expertise appropriate to evaluating specific NIOSH research programs and may include representatives of stakeholder groups (such as labor unions and industry) and experts in technology transfer and program evaluation. The committees will conduct appropriate information-gathering sessions to obtain information from the sponsor (a NIOSH research program), stakeholders affected directly by the NIOSH research, and relevant independent parties. Each EC will consist of about 10 members, will meet about three times, and will prepare a report. The National Academies will deliver the report to NIOSH within 9 months after the individual EC is formed. EC reports will be subjected to the National Academies report-review process.

I.D. Evaluation Committees' Information Needs

The ECs are expected to conduct information-gathering as appropriate on

- Background and resources of the program:
  - History of program, including results of previous reviews.
  - Program funding, by year, for the current year and the last 10 years.
  - Program funding, by objective or subprogram.
  - Extramural-grant awarding, cooperative agreement and contracting process, solicitation of research ideas, and advisory activities.
- Program goals and objectives.
- Internal NIOSH processes and research:
  - Intramural surveillance, research, and transfer activities.
  - Process to solicit and approve intramural research proposals.

---

[4]PART focuses on assessing program-level performance and is one of the measures of success for the Budget and Performance Integration initiative of the president's management agenda (see CDC Occupational Safety and Health at http://www.whitehouse.gov/omb/budget/fy2006/pma/hhs.pdf).

- NIOSH-funded extramural research:
  - Requests for proposals, cooperative agreements and research contracts distributed.
  - Awardee products, including close-out reports, surveillance, research, and transfer activities, peer-reviewed publications, and patents.
- Products and technology transfer:
  - Data related to program publications, conferences, recommendations, patents, and so on.
  - Past and planned mechanisms for transferring outputs to outcomes.
  - Interventions, recommendations, and information-dissemination and technology-transfer activities designed to get research findings used to improve occupational safety and health.
  - Outcomes of research, alerts, standard-setting, investigations, and consultations; for example—documented reductions in risk after program-supported interventions, employer and industry behavior changes made in response to research outputs, and worker behavior changes in response to research outputs.
- Impact on worker safety and health—data necessary to evaluate program impact on health outcomes (work-related injuries and illnesses) and exposures.
- The most severe or most frequent adverse health and safety outcomes or exposures in the research program and the most accessible improvements with respect to health and safety.
- Interactions within NIOSH and with other stakeholders:
  - The role of program research staff in NIOSH policy-setting, Occupational Safety and Health Administration (OSHA) and Mine Safety and Health Administration (MSHA) standard-setting, and voluntary standard-setting and other government policy functions.
  - Other institutions and research programs with overlapping or similar portfolios and an explanation of the relationship between the NIOSH work and staff and those of other institutions.
  - Stakeholder perspectives (OSHA, MSHA, union and workforce, industry, and so on).
  - Key partnerships with employers, labor, other government organizations, academic institutions, nonprofit organizations, and international organizations.
  - International involvement and perspective.
- Systems to identify emerging problems and emerging research, including plans.

II. SUMMARY OF EVALUATION PROCESS

The ECs are charged with assessing the relevance, quality, and impact of NIOSH research programs. In conducting their evaluations, the ECs should ascertain whether NIOSH is doing the right things (relevance) and doing them right (quality) and whether these things are improving health and safety in the workplace (impact).

II.A. The Evaluation Flow Chart (Figure 2)

To address its charges, the FC has developed a flow chart (Figure 2) that breaks the NIOSH logic model into discrete, sequential program components to be characterized or assessed by the ECs. The components to be assessed are as follows:

- Major program-area *challenges.*
- Strategic *goals and objectives.*
- *Inputs* (such as budget, staff, facilities, the institute's research management, the NIOSH Board of Scientific Counselors, the NORA process, and NORA work groups).
- *Activities* (efforts by NIOSH staff, contractors, and grantees, such as hazard and health-outcome surveillance, exposure-measurement research, health-effects research, intervention research, health services, other research, and technology-transfer activities).
- *Outputs* (the products of NIOSH activities, such as publications, reports, conferences, databases, tools, methods, guidelines, recommendations, education and training, and patents).
- *Intermediate outcomes* (responses by NIOSH stakeholders to NIOSH products, such as public or private policy change, training and education in the form of workshop or seminar attendance, self-reported use or repackaging of NIOSH data by intermediary stakeholders, adoption of technologies developed by NIOSH, implemented guidelines, licenses, and reduction of workplace hazardous exposures and other risk factors).
- *End outcomes* (such as reduction of work-related injuries or illnesses, or hazardous exposures in the workplace).

Drawing on the program logic model, the flow chart, and EC members' expertise, the ECs will delineate important determinants of a NIOSH research program's agenda and the consequences of the NIOSH research activity. Determinants are conceptualized as inputs and external factors. Examples of external factors are the research activities of industry and other federal agencies and the political and

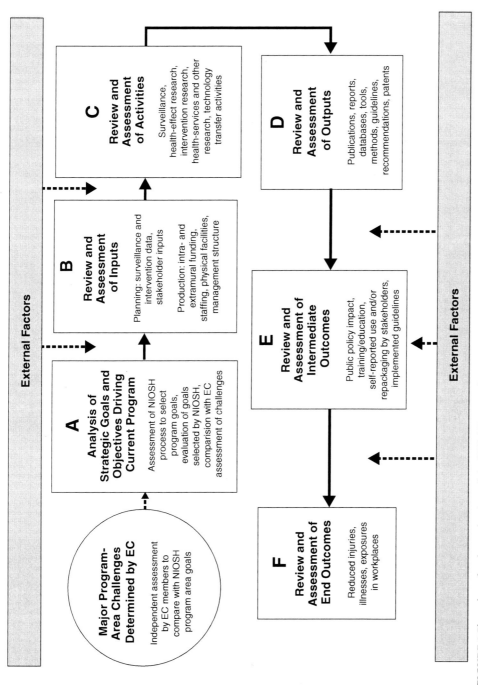

FIGURE 2 Flow chart for the evaluation of the NIOSH research program.

regulatory environment, which can affect all components of the research program (Figure 2). *For purposes of this review, the results of inputs and external factors are the program research activities, outputs, and associated transfer activities that may result in intermediate outcomes and possibly eventual end outcomes.*

The FC has used the NIOSH logic model to develop the flow chart to define the scope and steps of an EC evaluation. The FC's vision of how a program evaluation should occur is incorporated in a summary manner in the flow chart and discussed extensively in later sections. For example, the FC identified two types of outcomes: (a) *intermediate outcomes*, which represent implementations (what external stakeholders, such as employers, do in reaction to the products of NIOSH work, including new regulations, widely accepted guidelines, introduction of control technologies in the workplace, changes in employer or worker behaviors, and changes in diagnostic practices of health-care providers), and (b) *end outcomes*, which are improvements (reductions in work-related injuries, illnesses, and hazardous exposures). For the purpose of evaluation, the FC does not differentiate between NIOSH's "intermediate customer" and "final customer" activities (Figure 1); instead it combines them into a single category (Box E, Review and Assessment of Intermediate Outcomes, Figure 2). Training and development programs were appropriately defined as outputs by NIOSH in the logic model, but the FC finds more value in focusing on response to such offerings as intermediate outcomes (Box E) in the flow chart. The number of workers exposed to training activities represents a type of implementation of NIOSH outputs in the workplace. In evaluating each program or major subprogram, the EC must collect, analyze, and evaluate information on items described in each of the boxes of Figure 2. Further details on the evaluation are described in Section III of this document.

II.B. Steps in Program Evaluation

The FC has concluded that useful evaluation requires: (a) a disciplined focus on a small number of questions or hypotheses typically related to program goals, performance criteria, and performance standards; (b) a rigorous method for answering the questions or testing the hypotheses; and (c) a credible procedure for developing qualitative and quantitative assessments. The evaluation process developed by the FC is summarized here and described in detail in Section III of this document.

1. Gather appropriate information from NIOSH and other sources.
2. Determine timeframe that the evaluation will cover (see III.B.1).
3. Identify program-area major challenges and objectives (see III.B.2). All NIOSH research programs, whether based on health outcomes or sectors,

are designed to be responsive to the safety and health problems in today's or tomorrow's workplace. In the NIOSH vision, mission, values, and goals, each research program should have its own objectives. The ECs will provide an independent assessment of the major program challenges and determine whether they are consistent with the research program's stated goals and objectives.

4. Identify subprograms and major projects in the research program. It is important for each EC to determine how necessary it is to disaggregate a program to achieve a manageable and meaningful evaluation of its components and the total program. Each research program may need to be broken down into several recognizable subprograms or major projects if an effective evaluation is to be organized. It may be advantageous for an EC to disaggregate a program into subprograms that NIOSH identifies.
5. Evaluate the program and subprogram components sequentially as discussed in Section III, using the flow chart (Figure 2) as a guide (Sections III.B.3 through III.B.8). This will involve qualitatively assessing each phase of a research program by using the questions and guidance provided by the FC and professional judgment.
6. Evaluate the research program's potential outcomes not yet appreciated (Section III.B.9).
7. Evaluate and score the program outcomes and important subprogram outcomes specifically for contributions to improvements in workplace safety and health. A worksheet is provided with specific items for consideration (Section III.B.10).
8. Evaluate and score the overall program for impact (Section III.B.10). Final program ratings will consist of a numerical score and discussion of its rationale.
9. Evaluate and score the overall program for relevance (Section III.B.10). Final program ratings will consist of a numerical score and discussion of its rationale.
10. Identify significant emerging research areas (Section III.C). On the basis of the expert judgment of EC members and information gathered from stakeholders (such as labor, industry, academe, and government agencies) and from appropriate NIOSH sentinel-event field-investigation activities, the EC will respond to Charge 3 by identifying and describing emerging research that appears especially important in its relevance to the mission of NIOSH. The EC will assess the extent to which NIOSH's program is responsive to today's and tomorrow's needs and determine whether there are any gaps in response.
11. Prepare report by using the template provided in Section IV as a guide.

II.C. Assessing Relevance

FC members identified numerous *possible* factors to consider in assessing the relevance of NIOSH research programs, such as:

- The severity, frequency, or both of the health and safety outcomes addressed and the number of people at risk (magnitude) for these outcomes.
- The extent to which NIOSH research programs have identified and addressed gender issues and the concerns related to vulnerable populations. Vulnerable populations are defined as groups of workers who have (1) biological, social, or economic characteristics that place them at increased risk of developing work-related conditions and/or (2) inadequate data collected about them. Vulnerable populations include disadvantaged minorities, disabled individuals, low-wage workers, and non-English speakers for whom language or other barriers present health or safety risks.
- The extent to which NIOSH research programs have addressed the health and safety needs of small businesses.
- The "life stage" of the problems being addressed. As the health effects are understood, emphasis should shift to intervention research, and from efficacy to effectiveness to research on the process of dissemination of tested interventions. Gaps in the spectrum of prevention need to be addressed; for example, research on exposure assessment may be necessary before the next intervention steps can be taken.
- The structure, in addition to the content, of the research program. A relevant research program is more than a set of unrelated research projects; it is an integrated program involving an interrelated set of surveillance, research, and transfer activities.
- Appropriate consideration by NIOSH of stakeholder inputs.

II.D. Assessing Impact

Causal attribution is a major aspect of program evaluation. It is necessary for the ECs to assess, to the extent possible, NIOSH's contribution to end outcomes. Data on reductions in work-related injuries, illnesses, and hazardous exposures will be available for some programs. In some cases, they may be quantifiable. It is possible, however, to evaluate the impact of a NIOSH research program whether the outcomes are intermediate outcomes or end outcomes. Intermediate outcomes may be used as proxies for end outcomes in assessing impact if there is no direct evidence of improvements in health and safety as long as the ECs qualify their findings. The ECs will describe the realized or potential benefits of NIOSH's programs. Examples of realized intermediate outcomes include: new regulations, widely accepted guidelines, work practices, and procedures, all of which may contribute measurably to enhancing health and safety at the work place.

The contribution of a NIOSH program to technology now in use or being implemented is another important part of impact assessment. NIOSH's contribution can be assessed as major or important, moderate, likely, limited, or none. If technology development is in progress or has been abandoned, for whatever reason, the benefits are only potential or consist of knowledge gain.

III. EVALUATION OF NIOSH RESEARCH PROGRAMS—THE PROCESS

III.A. Analysis of External Factors Relevant to the NIOSH Research Program

As depicted in the logic model (Figure 1), the end outcome of reduced injuries, illnesses, or exposures is effected through stakeholder activities and outputs. All those involve the use of NIOSH outputs by stakeholders in industry, labor, other government agencies, and so on. It is evident that actions beyond NIOSH's control—by industry, labor, and other entities—have important bearings on the incorporation in the workplace of NIOSH's outputs to enhance health and safety. The implementation of research findings may depend on existing or future policy considerations.

III.A.1. Overview

External factors may be considered as forces beyond the control of NIOSH that may affect the evolution of the program. External factors dominate the evolution of the path from NIOSH inputs to occupational health and safety outcomes (Figure 1). External factors can also be considered inputs to the evaluation of each aspect (planning, implementation, transfer, and others) of NIOSH research programs (Figure 2).

Identification of external factors by the ECs is essential to providing a context for NIOSH program evaluation. External factors may best be assessed through the expert judgment of EC members regarding the knowledge base, the research program, and implementation of interventions as these relate to the needs in the occupational health or safety area targeted by the research program. The ECs, however, may choose additional approaches to assess external factors.

The FC recommends the ECs ask NIOSH to identify and describe external factors early in the evaluation sequence. Factors external to NIOSH might have been responsible for achieving some outcomes, and they might also have presented formidable obstacles. The ECs must address both possibilities.

III.A.2. Considerations for Discussion

Some external factors may involve constraints on research activity related to target populations, methodological issues, and resource availability. For example, evaluators might examine whether

- Projects addressing a critical health need are technologically feasible. A workforce with appropriate size and duration, magnitude, and distribution of exposure for measuring a health effect may not exist. For example, no population of workers has been exposed for 30 years to formaldehyde at the current OSHA Permissible Exposure Limit (PEL), so the related cancer mortality cannot yet be directly assessed.
- Research is inhibited because NIOSH investigators are unable to access an adequate study population. Under current policy, NIOSH must either obtain an invitation by management to study a workplace or seek a judicial order to provide authority to enter a worksite. (Cooperation under court order may well be insufficient for effective research.)
- Research is inhibited because the work environment, materials, and historical records cannot be accessed even with management and workforce cooperation.
- Adequate or established methods do not exist for assessing the environment.
- Records needed for historical-exposure reconstruction cannot be accessed or do not exist.
- Intervention research is inhibited because an appropriate employer partner cannot be identified to institute the intervention.
- The NIOSH contribution to a certain area of research is reduced because other institutions are working in the same area.
- NIOSH resources are inadequate to tackle the key questions.

Evaluation of the impact of NIOSH research outputs on outcomes may require consideration of external factors that might have impeded or aided implementation, measurement, and so on. For example, evaluators might consider whether

- Regulatory end points are unachievable because of obstacles to regulation or differing priorities of the regulatory agencies. For example, recommen-

dations for improved respiratory protection programs for health-care workers might not be implemented because of enforcement policies or lack of acceptance by the administration of health-care institutions.
- A feasible control for a known risk factor or exposure is not implemented because the costs of implementation are too high or the economic incentives under current circumstances do not favor such actions.
- Improvements in end points are unobservable because baseline and ongoing surveillance data are not available. For example, the current incidence of occupational noise-induced hearing loss is not known although surveillance for a significant threshold shift is feasible. (NIOSH conducts surveillance of work-related illnesses, injuries, and hazards, but comprehensive surveillance is not possible with existing resources.)
- Reductions in adverse effects of chronic exposure cannot be measured. For example, 90% of identified work-related mortality is from diseases, such as cancer, that arise only after decades of latency from first exposure; therefore, effects of reducing exposure to a carcinogen cannot be observed in the timeframe of most interventions.
- A regulation is promulgated that requires a technology that was developed but not widely used.

III.B. Evaluating NIOSH Research Programs (Addressing Charges 1 and 2)

III.B.1. Identifying Period of Time to Be Evaluated

Through study of materials presented by the NIOSH research program and other sources, an EC will become familiar with the history of the research program being evaluated and its major subprograms, program goals and objectives, resources, and other pertinent information.

It is useful for the ECs to consider three general timeframes in conducting their reviews:

- 1970-1995, the period from the founding of NIOSH to the initiation of the NORA process (pre-NORA period).
- 1996-2005 (NORA 1 period).
- Current period and forward (NORA 2 period).

It will be important for the ECs to get a general sense of the history of the NIOSH research program and its impact, but their efforts should be focused on the impact and relevance of NIOSH programs from 1996 on. It is recognized that many of the intermediate and end outcomes since 1996 are the consequence of research outputs accomplished earlier. Both the relevance of the research program targets of NORA 1 and the proposed NORA 2 objectives for the next decade should be considered.

NIOSH is in the midst of a substantial restructuring of the NORA agenda, and expert judgment about relevance and prospective impact of current research programs will be most useful to the agency. The timeframes provided here are only for general guidance; the exact dates of the period to focus on in reviewing programs will depend on the specific research program under review.

III.B.2. Identification of Major Challenges
(Circle in Figure 2)

Early in its assessment process, an EC should independently identify the major challenges for its research program. These would be the matters the EC believes should have priority in the research program being evaluated. In arriving at a list of challenges, the EC should rely on surveillance findings, including NIOSH investigations of sentinel events (through health-hazard or fatality-assessment programs), and its own expert judgment. Those should be supplemented with determinations or recommendations by appropriate advisory sources regardless of whether these sources have contributed to NIOSH program deliberations. This process will allow the EC to compare its assessment of challenges to be addressed by NIOSH with NIOSH program goals, and to evaluate the congruence between the two as a measure of relevance (Charge 2).

III.B.3. Analysis of Research Program Strategic Goals and Objectives
(Box A in Figure 2)

The research program goals and objectives should be evaluated, with a focus on how each research program's goals are related to NIOSH's agency-wide strategic goals and to the major current challenges and emerging problems identified in the step above. Differences may exist between the importance or relevance of an issue and the influence NIOSH-funded research might have in addressing the issue. The EC should recognize that NIOSH research priorities may be strategic rather than based on the assessment of the state of knowledge.

Some aspects of the NIOSH research program's strategic goals and objectives would have been already subjected to evaluation by internal or external bodies. Research program relevant evaluations that should be requested include the NIOSH annual program review by the Leadership Team; the NORA research program proposal pre-award external review, NORA post-award program external review, and external scientific program review.

Questions to Guide the Evaluation Committee

1. Are the strategic goals and objectives of the program well defined and clearly described?
2. In the last decade, how well were program goals and objectives aligned with NORA 1 priorities?
3. How do the current strategic goals and objectives of the program relate to the current NIOSH strategy, including NORA 2?
4. Are the research program goals, objectives, and strategies relevant to the major challenges in the research program and likely to address emerging problems in the research program (as determined by the EC)?
   a. Did past program goals and objectives (research and dissemination/transfer activities) focus on the most relevant problems and anticipate the emerging problems in the research program?
   b. Are the current program goals and objectives targeted to the most relevant problems and likely to address emerging problems in the research program?
5. How does the program identify emerging research areas?
   a. What information is reviewed by NIOSH?
   b. What advisory or stakeholder groups are asked to identify emerging areas?
   c. What new research areas have been identified in the program?
   d. Were important areas overlooked?

Assessment

The EC will provide a qualitative assessment discussing the relevance of the area's goals, objectives, and strategies as related to the research program's major challenges and emerging problems.

III.B.4. Review of Inputs
(Box B in Figure 2)

Inputs are categorized as planning or production inputs in the NIOSH logic model. Planning inputs include stakeholder inputs, surveillance and intervention data, and risk assessments. Production inputs include intramural and extramural funding, staffing, management structure, and physical facilities.

Inputs for program evaluation include existing intramural and extramural information and, potentially, surveys or case studies that might have been developed specifically to assess progress in reducing workplace illnesses and injuries and to provide information relevant to targeting research appropriately to future needs. The ECs should request the relevant planning and production inputs from NIOSH.

Planning Inputs

Planning inputs can be qualitative or quantitative. Sources of qualitative inputs include

- Federal Advisory Committee Act panels (Board of Scientific Counselors, Mine Safety and Health Research Advisory Committee, National Advisory Committee on Occupational Safety and Health, and so on).
- NORA research partners, initial NORA stakeholder meetings, later NORA Team efforts (especially strategic research plans), and the NORA Liaison Committee and federal liaison committee recommendations.
- Other federal research agendas, industry, labor, academe, professional associations, industry associations, and Council of State and Territorial Epidemiologists.
- OSHA and MSHA strategic plans.

Attention should be given to how comprehensive the inputs have been and to what extent gaps have been identified or considered.

Sources of quantitative inputs include

- Intramural surveillance information, such as descriptive data on exposures and outcomes (appropriate data may be available from a number of NIOSH divisions and laboratories).
- Health Hazard Evaluations (HHEs).
- Reports from the Fatality Assessment Control and Evaluation (FACE) program.
- Extramural health-outcome and exposure-assessment data from (1) OSHA and MSHA (inspection data) and the Bureau of Labor Statistics, U.S. Department of Defense, and U.S. Department of Agriculture (fatality, injury, and illness surveillance data); (2) state government partners, including NIOSH-funded state surveillance programs, such as Sentinel Event Notification System of Occupational Risks (SENSOR), Adult Blood

Lead Epidemiology and Surveillance (ABLES), and state-based FACE; and (3) non-government organizations, such as the Association of Occupational and Environmental Clinics (AOEC) and the American College of Occupational and Environmental Medicine (ACOEM).
- Appropriate data from NIOSH-funded, investigator-initiated extramural research.

Production Inputs

For each research program under review, NIOSH should specify an identifiable portion of the NIOSH intramural budget, staff, facilities, and management that has been allocated by divisions and offices that play a major role in the research program. Production inputs should be described primarily in terms of intramural research projects and staff, relevant extramural projects (particularly cooperative agreements and contracts), and HHEs and related staff. Consideration should also be given to budget inputs for program evaluation and to leveraged funds provided by partners, such as National Institutes of Health and the Environmental Protection Agency joint requests for applications or program announcements and OSHA, MSHA, and Department of Defense contracts with NIOSH to conduct work.

Assessment of those inputs should include consideration of (1) the degree to which allocation of funding and personnel has been reasonably consistent with the resources needed to conduct the research and (2) the extent to which funding for the relevant intramural research program activity has been limited by lack of discretionary spending beyond salaries (travel, supplies, external laboratory services, and so on). The assessments, therefore, should consider the adequacy of the qualitative and quantitative planning inputs and the use and adequacy of production inputs, particularly (1) and (2) above.

Questions as a Guide for the Evaluation Committee

1. Were the planning, production, and other input data adequate?
2. How well were the major planning, production, and other program inputs used to promote the major activities?
3. Were the sources of inputs and the amount and quality of inputs adequate?
4. Was input obtained from stakeholders representing vulnerable working populations and small businesses?
5. Were production inputs (intramural and extramural funding, staffing, management, and physical infrastructure resources) consistent with goals and objectives of the program?

Assessment

The EC will provide a qualitative assessment that discusses the quality, adequacy, and use of inputs.

III.B.5. Review of Activities
(Box C in Figure 2)

Activities are defined as the efforts and work of the program, its staff, and its grantees and contractors. For purposes of the present evaluation, activities of the NIOSH program under review should be divided into research and transfer activities. Research activities may be further categorized as surveillance, health-effects research, intervention research, health-services research, and other research (see sample classification of research activities in Table 2). Transfer activities include information dissemination, training, technical assistance, and education designed to translate research outputs into content and formats designed for application in the workplace to produce improvements in occupational safety and health. Depending on the scope of the program under review, activities may also be grouped by research program objectives or subprograms.

Conventional occupational-health research focuses appropriately on health effects and technology. A focus on socioeconomic and policy research and on surveillance and diffusion research is also needed to effect change because not all relevant intermediate outcomes occur in the workplace. There are important outcomes farther out on the causal chain that NIOSH can affect and thereby influence health and safety in the workplace. Some examples of types of research that might also prove important in addressing NIOSH's mission are

- Socioeconomic research on cost shifting between worker compensation and private insurance.
- Surveillance research to assess the degree of significant and systematic underreporting of select injuries and illnesses on OSHA logs.
- Research on methods to build health and safety capacity in community health centers that serve low-income and/or minority-group workers, and to improve recognition and treatment of work-related conditions.
- Transfer research to change health and safety knowledge in teenagers while they are in high school to improve the likelihood of reduced injuries when they enter the workforce.
- Community-based participatory research on differences between recently arrived immigrants and US-born workers regarding perceptions of acceptable health and safety risks to target programs to meet the workforce training needs of immigrant workers.

Appendix A

TABLE 2 Examples of NIOSH Program Research and Transfer Activities

Surveillance
(including hazard and health surveillance and evaluation of surveillance systems)

Health-effects research
Epidemiologic research
Toxicologic research
Laboratory-based physical and safety risk factor research
Development of clinical screening methods and tools

Exposure-assessment research
Intervention research
Control technology
    Engineering controls and alternatives
    Administrative controls
    Personal protective equipment
Work organization research
Community-based participatory research
Policy research (such as alternative approaches to targeting inspections)
Diffusion and dissemination research
    Training effectiveness
    Information-dissemination effectiveness
    Diffusion of technology

Health-services and other research
    Access to occupational health care
    Infrastructure research—delivery of occupational-health services, including international health and safety
    Socioeconomic consequences of work-related injuries and illnesses
    Worker compensation

Technology-transfer and other transfer activities
    Information dissemination
    Training programs

The ECs should review the list of research and transfer activities (projects) for the research program under review that have been completed, are in progress, or have been planned. Surveillance activities should be included in this review. An EC should request that the NIOSH program under review provide a list of activities, grouping the projects into research activities as in Table 2, and specify whether they are intramural or extramural. For extramural projects, the key organizations and principal investigators' names should be requested, as should whether the projects were in response to a request for proposal or a request for application. For an intramural project, the EC should ask NIOSH to provide a list of key collaborators (other government agency, academe, industry, and/or union partners).

The ECs should evaluate each of the research activities outlined in Table 2 to the extent that each forms an important element of the program research. In the case of a sector research program (for example, mining, construction) in which health-effects research is not being reviewed, the ECs should determine what research inputs are being used by the program to develop its targets and then assess the value of the inputs.

Questions to Guide the Evaluation Committee in Assessing Research Activities

1. What are the major subprograms or groupings of activities within the program?
2. Were the activities consistent with program goals and objectives?
3. Were the research activities relevant to the major challenges in the research program?
    a. Did they address the most serious outcomes?
    b. Did they address the most common outcomes?
    c. Did they address the needs of both genders, vulnerable working populations, and small businesses?
4. Were the research activities appropriately responsive to the input of stakeholders?
5. To what extent were partners involved in the research activities?
6. Are the resource allocations appropriate, and appropriate at this time, for the research activities?
7. To what extent did peer reviews (internal, external, and precourse or midcourse) affect the activities?
8. Is there adequate monitoring of quality assurance procedures to ensure credible research data, analyses, and conclusions?

Questions to Guide the Evaluation Committee in Assessing Transfer Activities

1. Is there a coherent planned program of transfer activities?
2. Are the program's information dissemination, training, education, technical assistance, or publications successful in reaching the workplace or relevant stakeholders in other settings? How widespread is the response?
3. To what extent did the program build research and education capacity (internal or external)?

Assessment

For this part of the assessment, the EC will provide a qualitative assessment discussing relevance and quality. This evaluation must include consideration of the external factors identified in Section III.A that constrain choices of research projects. The EC will consider the appropriateness of resource allocations with respect to issues' importance and the extent to which the issue is being addressed. A highly relevant and high-quality program would be comprehensive, address high-priority needs, produce high-quality results, be highly collaborative, and be of value to stakeholders. Programs may be progressively less relevant or of lower quality as those key elements are not up to the mark or are missing. The discussion should cover those aspects in sufficient detail to arrive at a qualitative assessment of the activities. Assessment of the transfer activities must include considerations of program planning, coherence, quality, and impact.

III.B.6. Review of Outputs
(Box D in Figure 2)

As shown in Figure 1, research inputs and activities lead to outputs. An output is a direct product of a NIOSH research program that is logically related to the achievement of desirable and intended outcomes. Outputs are created for researchers, practitioners, intermediaries, and end-users, such as consumers. Outputs can be in the form of publications in peer-reviewed journals, recommendations, reports, Web-site content, workshops and presentations, databases, educational materials, scales and methods, new technologies, patents, technical assistance, and so on. Outputs of NIOSH's extramurally funded activities should also be considered. Examples of major outputs are provided in Table 3.

Depending on the intended audience, outputs may be tailored to communicate information most effectively to increase the likelihood of comprehension, knowledge, attitude formation, and behavioral intent. The extent of use of formative evaluation data (data gathered prior to communication for the purpose of improving the likelihood of the intended effects) or intended user feedback in the design of the output can be considered an indicator of output quality.

In addition to outputs themselves, many related indicators of the production, reference to, and utility of outputs can be conceptualized and made operational. Examples include the extent of collaboration with other organizations in the determination of research agendas, the conduct of research, the dissemination of research results, and interorganizational involvement in the production of outputs. Coauthorship is a measure of the centrality of NIOSH researchers in the broader research community.

TABLE 3 Examples of a Variety of Scientific Information Outputs

Peer-reviewed publications by NIOSH staff
Total number of original research articles by NIOSH staff
Total number of review articles by NIOSH staff (including best-practice articles)
Complete citation for each written publication
Complete copies of the "top five" articles
Collaboration with other public- or private-sector researchers
Publications in the field of interest with other support by investigators also funded by NIOSH (for example, ergonomic studies with other support by an investigator funded by NIOSH to do ergonomics work, in which case NIOSH should get some credit for seeding interest or drawing people into the field)

Peer-reviewed publications by external researchers funded by NIOSH
Total number of NIOSH-funded original research articles by external researchers
Total number of NIOSH-funded review articles by external researchers (including best-practices articles)
Complete citation for each written report
Complete copies of the "top five" articles
Collaboration with other government or academic researchers

NIOSH reports in the research program
Total number of written reports
Complete citation for each written report
Complete copies of the "top five" reports

Sponsored conferences and workshops
Total number of sponsored conferences
Total number of sponsored workshops
For each sponsored conference or workshop, describe:
    Title, date, and location
    Partial vs complete sponsorship (if partial, who were cosponsors?)
    Approximate number of attendees and composition of participants
    Primary "products" of the event (such as publication of conference proceedings)
NIOSH's assessment of value or impact

Databases
Total number of major databases created by NIOSH staff
Total number of major databases created by external researchers funded by NIOSH grants,
For each database:
    Title, objective (in one to four sentences), and start and stop dates
    Partial vs complete sponsorship (if partial, who were cosponsors?)
    Study or surveillance-system design, study population, and sample size
    Primary "products" of the database (such as number of peer-reviewed articles and reports)
    Complete copies of the "top two" publications and/or findings, to date, from each database

APPENDIX A

TABLE 3 Continued

Recommendations
Total number of major recommendations
For each:
　Complete citation (article, report, or conference where recommendation was made)
　Summary in one to four sentences
　Percentage of target audience that has adopted recommendation 1, 5, and 10 years later
　Up to three examples of implementation in the field
Identifications of "top five" recommendations to date

Tools, methods, or technologies (TMT)
Total number of major TMT (includes training and education materials)
For each:
　Title and objective of TMT (in one to four sentences)
　Complete citation (if applicable)
　Percentage of target audience that has used TMT 1, 5, and 10 years later
　Up to three examples of implementation in the field
Identification of "top five" TMT to date

Patents
Total number of patents
For each:
　Title and objective patent (in one to four sentences)
　Complete citation
　Percentage of target audience that has used product 1, 5, and 10 years later
　Up to three examples of implementation in the field
Identification of "top five" patents to date

Miscellaneous
Any other important program outputs

　　The EC should ask NIOSH to provide information on all relevant outputs for the specific program for the chosen time period.

Questions to Guide the Evaluation Committee

1. What are the major outputs of the research program?
2. Did the research program produce outputs that addressed the high-priority areas?
3. To what extent did the program generate important new knowledge or technology?

4. Are there peer-reviewed publications that are widely cited and considered to report "breakthrough" results?
5. Were outputs relevant to both genders, vulnerable populations, and health disparities?
6. Were outputs relevant to health and safety problems of small businesses?
7. Are products user-friendly in terms of readability, simplicity, and design?
8. To what extent did the program help to build the internal or extramural institutional knowledge base?
9. Did the research produce effective cross-agency, cross-institute, or internal-external collaborations?

Assessment

For this part of the assessment, the EC should provide a qualitative assessment discussing relevance, quality, and usefulness. A highly ranked program will be one with outputs that address needs in high-priority areas, contain new knowledge or technology that is effectively communicated, contribute to capacity-building both inside and outside NIOSH, and are relevant to the pertinent populations. The discussion should cover those aspects in sufficient detail to support the qualitative assessment of the outputs.

III.B.7. Review of Intermediate Outcomes (Box E in Figure 2)

Intermediate outcomes, for the purposes of this evaluation, are related to the program's association with behaviors and changes at individual, group, and organizational levels in the workplace. An intermediate outcome reflects an assessment of worth by stakeholders outside NIOSH (such as managers in industrial firms) about NIOSH research or its products.

Intermediate outcomes include the production of standards, or regulations based in whole or in part on NIOSH research (products adopted as public policy or as policy or guidelines by private organizations or industry); attendance at training and education programs sponsored by other organizations; use of publications by workers, industry, and occupational safety and health professionals in the field; and citations of NIOSH research by industrial and academic scientists.

More difficult-to-collect intermediate outcomes that may be valid indicators of quality or utility include self-report measures by users and relevant nonusers of NIOSH outputs. These indicators include the extent to which key intermediaries find value in NIOSH databases for the repackaging of health and safety information, the extent to which NIOSH recommendations are in place and attended to in workplaces, and employee or employer knowledge of and adherence to NIOSH-recommended practices.

A research program might be evaluated in terms of whether it is recognized as a national center of excellence, is one of the larger and best research programs in the country, is recognized only in terms of particular staff or a particular laboratory, duplicates other, larger facilities, or is not unique or has little capability or capacity.

Questions to Guide the Evaluation Committee

1. Has the program resulted in stakeholder training or education activities that are being used in the workplace or in school or apprentice programs? If so, what is the response to what is being done, and how widespread is the response?
2. Has the program resulted in standards, regulations, public policy, or voluntary guidelines that have been transferred to or created by the workplace in response to NIOSH outputs?
3. Has the program resulted in new control technology or administrative control concepts that are feasible for use or have been adopted in the workplace to reduce risk factors?
4. Has the program resulted in new personal protective equipment that is feasible for use or has been adopted in the workplace to reduce risk factors or exposures?
5. Has the program contributed to changes in health care practices to improve recognition and management of occupational health conditions?
6. Has the program resulted in research partnerships with stakeholders leading to changes in the workplace?
7. To what extent did the program's stakeholders find value in NIOSH's products (as shown by document requests, web hits, conference attendance, and so on)?
8. Has the program resulted in changes in employer or worker practices associated with the reduction of risk factors?
9. Does the program or a subprogram provide unique staff or laboratory capability that is a necessary national resource? If so, is it adequate or does it need to be enhanced or reduced?
10. Has the program resulted in interventions that protect both genders, vulnerable workers or address the needs of small businesses?
11. To what extent did the program contribute to increased capacity at worksites to identify or respond to threats to safety and health?

Assessment

Only a qualitative assessment of product development, usefulness, and impact is required at this point in the EC report. Some thought should be given to the relative value of intermediate outcomes, and the FC recommends applying the well-accepted hierarchy-of-controls model. The discussion could include comments on how widely products have been used or programs implemented. The qualitative discussion should be specific as to the various products developed by the program and the extent of their use by specific entities (industry, labor, government, and so on) for specific purposes. Whether the products have resulted in changes in the workplace or in the reduction of risk factors should be discussed. The recognition accorded to the program or the facilities by its peers (such as recognition as a "center of excellence" by national and international communities) should be considered in the assessment. A program to be highly ranked should have a high level of performance in most of the relevant questions in this section. Whether the impact was caused by NIOSH alone or in combination with external agents should also be considered in the evaluation. An aspect of the evaluation can be whether the impact would have probably occurred without NIOSH's efforts.

III.B.8. Review of End Outcomes
(Box F in Figure 2)

End outcomes are defined by measures of health and safety and of impact on process and programs. The FC recognizes that a major challenge in assessing the causal relationship between NIOSH research and specific occupational health and safety outcomes is that NIOSH does not have direct responsibility or authority for implementing its research findings in the workplace. Furthermore, the benefits of NIOSH research program outputs can be realized, potential, or limited to knowledge gain. For example, negative studies contribute to the knowledge base and the generation of important new knowledge is a recognized form of outcome, in the absence of measurable impacts.

Outcome impact depends on there being a "receptor" for research results, including regulatory agencies, consensus and professional organizations, and employers. The ECs should consider questions related to the various stages that lead to outputs, such as

1. Did NIOSH research identify a gap in protection or a means of reduction of risk?
2. Did NIOSH convey that information to potential users in a usable form?
3. Was the research applied?
4. Did the results work?

APPENDIX A

End outcomes, for purposes of this evaluation, are changes related to health, including decreases in injuries, illnesses, deaths, and decreases in exposures or risk factors resulting from the research in the specific program or subprogram. Quantitative data are preferable to qualitative, but qualitative analysis may be necessary.

Sources of quantitative data include

- Bureau of Labor Statistics (BLS) data on fatal occupational injuries (Census of Fatal Occupational Injuries) and nonfatal injuries and illnesses (Annual Survey of Occupational Injury and Illnesses).
- NIOSH intramural surveillance systems, such as the National Electronic Injury Surveillance System (NEISS), the coal worker x-ray surveillance program, and agricultural worker surveys conducted by NIOSH in collaboration with the US Department of Agriculture.
- State-based surveillance systems, such as the NIOSH-funded ABLES, and the SENSOR programs (for asthma, pesticides, silicosis, noise-induced hearing loss, dermatitis, and burns).
- Selected state workers-compensation programs.
- OSHA, which collects exposure data, in the Integrated Management Information System.

The FC is unaware of surveillance mechanisms for many occupationally related chronic illnesses such as cancers arising from long exposure to chemicals and other stressors. For many outcomes, incidence and prevalence are best evaluated by investigator-initiated research.

The strengths and weaknesses of the various sources of outcome data should be recognized by the ECs. Quantitative accident, injury, illness, and employment data and databases are subject to error and bias and should be used by the ECs for drawing inferences only after critical evaluation and examination of whatever corroborating data are available. For example, it is widely recognized that occupational illnesses are poorly documented in the BLS Survey of Occupational Injuries and Illnesses, which captures only incident cases among active workers. Most illnesses that may have a relationship to work are not exclusively so related, and it is difficult for health practitioners to diagnose work-relatedness; few are adequately trained to make this assessment. Many of these illnesses have long latency and do not appear until years after people have left the employment in question. Surveillance programs may systematically undercount some categories of workers, such as contingent workers. Challenges posed by inadequate or inaccurate measurement systems should not drive programs out of difficult areas of study, and the ECs will need to be aware of such a possibility. In particular, contingent and informal working arrangements that place workers at greatest risk are also those on which surveillance information is almost totally lacking, so novel methods for measuring impact may be required.

In addition to measures of illness and injury, levels of exposure to chemical and physical agents and to safety and ergonomic hazards can be useful. Exposure or probability of exposure can serve as an appropriate proxy for disease or injury when a well-described occupational exposure-health association exists. In such instances, decreased exposure can be accepted as evidence that the end outcome of reduced illness has been achieved. That is particularly necessary in cases (such as exposure to asbestos) in which latency between exposure and disease outcome (lung cancer) makes effective evaluation of the relevant end outcome infeasible.

As an example of how exposure levels can serve as a proxy, the number of sites that exceed an OSHA Permissible Exposure Limit (PEL) or an American Conference of Governmental Industrial Hygienists threshold limit value is a quantitative measure of improvement of occupational health awareness and reduction of risk. In addition to exposure level, the number of people exposed and the distribution of exposure levels are important. Those data are available from multiple databases and studies of exposure. Apart from air monitoring, such measures of exposure as biohazard controls, reduction in requirements for use of personal protective equipment, and reduction of ergonomic risks are important.

Clearly, the commitment of industry, labor, and government to health and safety are critical external factors. Several measures of this commitment can be useful for the EC: monetary commitment of the groups, attitude, staffing, and surveys of relative level of importance. To the extent that the resources allocated to safety and health are limiting factors, the ECs should explicitly assess NIOSH performance in the context of constraints.

Questions to Guide the Evaluation Committee

1. What are the amounts and qualities of end-outcomes data (such as injuries, illness, exposure and productivity affected by health)?
2. What is the temporal trend in those data?
3. Is there objective evidence of improvements in occupational safety or health?
4. To what degree has the NIOSH program or subprogram been responsible for improvements in occupational safety or health?
5. If there is no time trend in the data, how do findings compare with data from other comparable US groups or the corresponding populations in other countries?
6. Is there evidence that external factors have affected outcome measures?
7. Has the program been responsible for outcomes outside the United States that have not been described in another category?

Assessment

For this part of the assessment, the EC should provide a qualitative assessment discussing the evidence of reductions in injuries and illnesses or their appropriate proxies (impacts).

III.B.9. Review of Other Outcomes

There may be health and safety impacts not yet appreciated, and other beneficial social, economic, and environmental outputs, including potential NIOSH impacts outside the United States. Many NIOSH study results and training programs may be judged to be important, or there may be evidence of implementation of NIOSH recommendations, outside the United States.

Questions to Guide the Evaluation Committee

1. Is the program likely to produce a favorable change that has not yet occurred or not been appreciated?
2. Has the program been responsible for other social, economic, security, or environmental outcomes?
3. Has the program's work had an impact on occupational health and safety in other countries?

Assessment

Evaluation by the EC may consist of a discussion of other outcomes, including positive changes that have not yet occurred; other social, economic, security, or environmental outcomes; and the impact that NIOSH has had on international occupational safety and health. It might also consider the incorporation of international research results into the NIOSH program of knowledge transfer for industry sectors.

III.B.10. Summary Evaluation Ratings and Rationale

An EC should use its expert judgment to rate the relevance and impact of the research program and its important subprograms by first summarizing its assessments of the subprograms and overall program according to the several items listed in Table 4. Table 4 is only a *worksheet* intended as an aid to the EC in its evaluation. Its purpose is to encourage the EC to summarize its work in one place and to concentrate on the subprograms and the items that will contribute to the final impact and relevance scores.

TABLE 4 Evaluation Committee Worksheet to Assess Research Programs and Subprograms
Please respond to each with "major or important," "moderate," "likely," "limited," or "none."

Background Context for Program Impact
1.1 Evidence of reduction of risk factors in the workplace (intermediate outcome) and evidence that external factors affected reduction
1.2 Evidence of reduction in workplace exposure, illness, or injuries (end outcome) and evidence that external factors affected reduction

			Subprogram			
Addressing Charge 1	Activity Category	Program	1	…	…	n
1.3 Contributions of NIOSH research and transfer activities to changes in work-related practices	Research					
	Transfer					
1.4 Contributions of NIOSH research and transfer activities to reductions in workplace exposure, illness, or injuries	Research					
	Transfer					
1.5 Evidence of external factors preventing application of NIOSH research results	Research					
	Transfer					
1.6 Contribution of NIOSH research to enhancement of capacity in government or other research institutions	Research					
	Transfer					
1.7 Contributions of NIOSH research to productivity, security, or environmental quality (beneficial side effects)	Research					
	Transfer					
Addressing Charge 2						
2.1 Relevance of current and recently completed research and transfer activities to future improvements in workplace safety and health	Research					
	Transfer					
2.2 Progress in targeting research to areas of study most relevant to future improvements in occupational safety and health	Research					
	Transfer					

To set the context for this step in the evaluation of the impact of the research program in preparation to respond to charge 1, the EC will first need to consider the available evidence of changes in work-related risks and adverse effects and external factors related to the changes. That information should be organized as a prose response to items 1.1 and 1.2 in Table 4.

Next, the EC should review the responses to the questions in Sections III.B.6 through III.B.8 and systematically rate the impact of the research program and its subprograms by responding to items 1.3-1.7 in Table 4. To complete the table, the EC response should use one of the following five terms: "major or important," "moderate," "likely," "limited," or "none" (since 1995). The EC should evaluate separately the impact of the research and the impact of transfer activities. High ratings on items 1.3-1.7 require the committee's judgment that the program has contributed to outcomes. For example, outcomes have occurred earlier than they would have or are better than they would have been in the absence of the research program, or outcomes would have occurred in the absence of external factors beyond NIOSH's control or ability to plan around.

The EC should then assess the relevance of the research program and subprograms in preparation for addressing charge 2. The EC should review the responses to the questions in Sections III.B.2 through III.B.5 and rate the relevance of the research program and its subprograms by responding to items 2.1 and 2.2 in Table 4. The same five terms should be used ("major or important," "moderate," "likely," "limited," or "none") to evaluate separately the relevance of the research and the relevance of the transfer activities. Transfer activities occur in two contexts: (1) NIOSH efforts to translate intellectual products into practice and (2) efforts by stakeholders to take advantage of NIOSH products.

Final Program Ratings

To provide the final assessment of the research program for charge 1 (impact) and charge 2 (relevance), the ECs will use their expert judgment, their responses to the questions in Table 4, and any other appropriate information to arrive at one overall rating for the impact of the research program and one for its relevance to the improvement of occupational safety and health. In light of substantial differences among the types of research programs that will be reviewed and the challenge to arrive at a summative evaluation of both impact and relevance, however, the FC chose not to attempt to construct a single algorithm to produce the two final ratings.

Having completed Table 4, the EC should undertake its final assessment of the impact and relevance of the program. Final program ratings will consist of the numerical scores and prose descriptions of why the scores were given. As explained below, the ECs will summarize their responses to charges 1 and 2 by rating the relevance and impact of the NIOSH research program on five-point scales in which 1 is the lowest and 5 the highest rating. The FC has made an effort to establish mutually exclusive rating categories in the five-point rating scale; when the basis of a rating fits more than one category, the highest applicable score should be assigned. ECs will need to consider the impact and relevance of both NIOSH completed research and research in progress. In general, the assessment of impact will consider research completed, and the assessment of relevance will include research in progress related to likely future improvements. When assessing the relevance of the program, the EC should keep in mind how well the program has considered the frequency and severity of the problems being addressed, whether appropriate attention has been directed to both genders, vulnerable populations or hard-to-reach workplaces, and whether the different needs of large and small businesses have been accounted for.

The FC has some concern that the impact scoring system proposed below might be considered a promotion of the conventional occupational-health research paradigm that focuses on health-effect and technology research and not give much emphasis to socioeconomic and policy research and to surveillance and diffusion research (as opposed to activities) needed to effect change. Clearly, not all intermediate outcomes occur in the workplace. There are important outcomes much farther out on the causal chain that NIOSH can affect, and not all these can be defined as well-accepted intermediate outcomes. NIOSH, for example, has an important role to play in generating knowledge that may contribute to changing norms in the insurance industry, in health-care practice, in public-health practice, and in the community at large. The ECs may find that some of these issues need to be addressed and considered as important to influence the external factors that limit application of more traditional research findings. Given the rapidly changing nature of work and the workforce and some of the intractable problems in manufacturing, mining, and some other fields, the ECs are encouraged to think beyond the traditional paradigm.

Rating of Impact

- 5 = Research program has made a major contribution to worker health and safety on the basis of end outcomes or well-accepted intermediate outcomes.
- 4 = Research program has made a moderate contribution on the basis of end outcomes or well-accepted intermediate outcomes; research program generated important new knowledge and is engaged in transfer activities, but well-accepted intermediate outcomes or end outcomes have not been documented.

3 = Research program activities or outputs are going on and are likely to produce improvements in worker health and safety (with explanation of why not rated higher).
2 = Research program activities or outputs are going on and may result in new knowledge or technology, but only limited application is expected.
1 = Research activities and outputs are NOT likely to have any application.
NA = Impact cannot be assessed; program not mature enough.

Rating of Relevance

5 = Research is in highest-priority subject areas and highly relevant to improvements in workplace protection; research results in, and NIOSH is engaged in, transfer activities at a significant level (highest rating).
4 = Research is in high-priority subject area and adequately connected to improvements in workplace protection; research results in, and NIOSH is engaged in, transfer activities.
3 = Research focuses on lesser priorities and is loosely or only indirectly connected to workplace protection; NIOSH is not significantly involved in transfer activities.
2 = Research program is not well integrated or well focused on priorities and is not clearly connected to workplace protection and inadequately connected to transfer activities.
1 = Research in the research program is an ad hoc collection of projects, is not integrated into a program, and is not likely to improve workplace safety or health.

III.C. Identifying Significant Emerging Research (Addressing Charge 3)

Among the most challenging aspects of conducting research for the purpose of prevention of injury and illness is identifying new or emerging needs or trends and formulating an active research response that appropriately uses scarce resources in anticipation of those needs. Each EC should review the procedures that NIOSH has in place to identify needed research relevant to the NIOSH mission.

Each EC should review the success that NIOSH has had in identifying and addressing research to emerging issues. The review should include examination of leading indicators from appropriate federal agency sources, such as the Environmental Protection Agency, the Department of Labor, the National Institute of Standards and Technology, the National Institutes of Health, the Department of Defense, and the Department of Commerce. Those indicators should track new technologies, products, and processes and disease or injury trends.

One source of inputs deserving particular attention is the NIOSH HHE reports. NIOSH's HHE program is a separate legislatively mandated program that offers a potential mechanism to identify emerging research needs that could be incorporated as an input in each of the programs evaluated. The ECs should consider whether appropriate consideration has been given to findings from the HHE investigations as they are related to the research program under review.

Some additional indicators might include NIOSH and the NIOSH-funded FACE, the AOEC reports, the US Chemical Safety Board investigations, SENSOR and other state-based surveillance programs, and others. In addition, appropriate federal advisory committees and other stakeholder groups should be consulted to provide qualitative information.

The EC members should use their expert judgment both to evaluate what NIOSH has identified as emerging research targets (charge 2) and to respond to charge 3 by providing recommendations to NIOSH for additional research that NIOSH has not yet identified. An EC's response to charge 3 will consist primarily of recommendations for research in subjects that the EC considers important and of the committee's rationale.

Questions to Guide the Evaluation Committee

1. What information does NIOSH review to identify emerging research needs?
    a. What is the process for review?
    b. How often does the process take place?
    c. How are NIOSH staff scientists and NIOSH leadership engaged?
    d. What is the process for moving from ideas to formal planning and resource allocation?
2. How are stakeholders involved?
    a. What advisory or stakeholder groups are asked to identify emerging research targets?
    b. How often are such groups consulted, and how are suggestions followed up?
3. What new research targets have been identified for future development in the program under evaluation?
    a. How were they identified?
    b. Were there lessons learned that could help to identify other emerging issues?
    c. Does the EC agree with the issues identified and selected as significant and with the NIOSH response, or were important issues overlooked?
    d. Is there evidence of unwise expenditure of resources on unimportant issues?

APPENDIX A

IV. EVALUATION COMMITTEE REPORT TEMPLATE

The following outline flows from the FC's review of the generalized logic model prepared by NIOSH, the request for information from NIOSH programs, and the assessment model described earlier in this report.

I. **Introduction:**
   This section should be a brief descriptive summary of the history of the program (and subprograms) being evaluated, with respect to pre-NORA, NORA 1, and current and future plans of the research program presented by NIOSH. It presents the context for the research on safety and health; goals, objectives, and resources; groupings of subprograms; and any other significant or pertinent information. (A list of the NIOSH materials reviewed should be provided in an appendix to the EC report.)

II. **Evaluation of programs and subprograms (charges 1 and 2):**
   A. Evaluation summary (includes a brief summary of the evaluation with respect to impact and relevance, scores for impact and relevance, and summary statements addressing charges 1 and 2).
   B. Strategic goals and objectives: Describes assessment of the subprograms and overall program for relevance.
   C. Review of inputs: Describes adequacy of inputs to achieve goals.
   D. Review of activities: Describes assessment of the relevance and quality of the activities.
   E. Review of research program outputs: Describes assessment of relevance, quality, and potential usefulness of the research program.
   F. Review of intermediate outcomes and causal impact: Describes assessment of the intermediate outcomes and the causal attribution to NIOSH; includes the likely impacts and recent outcomes in the assessment.
   G. Review of end outcomes: Describes the end outcomes related to health and safety and provides an assessment of the type and degree of causal attribution to NIOSH.
   H. Review of other outcomes: Discusses other health and safety impacts that have not yet occurred; other beneficial social, economic, and environmental outcomes; and international dimensions and outcomes.
   I. Summary of ratings and rationale (see Table 4).

III. Identification of needed research (charge 2):
The EC should assess the progress that the NIOSH program has made in targeting new research in the fields of occupational safety and health. There should be a discussion of the assessment process and results.

IV. Emerging research areas (charge 3):
The EC should assess whether the NIOSH program has identified significant emerging research areas that appear especially important in terms of their relevance to the mission of NIOSH. The EC should respond to NIOSH's perspective and add its own recommendations.

V. Recommendations for program improvement:
On the basis of the review and evaluation of the program, the EC may provide recommendations for improving the relevance of the NIOSH research program to health and safety conditions in the workplace and the impact of the research program on health and safety in the workplace as related to the research program under review.

Appendix A: List of the NIOSH and related materials collected in the process of the evaluation.

V. FRAMEWORK COMMITTEE FINAL REPORT

At the conclusion of all individual program reviews, the FC will prepare a final report summarizing the findings of all the evaluating committees and providing NIOSH with an overall evaluation. All program ratings will be summarized and might be plotted graphically or with a Web chart.

The following is a proposed outline of the FC's final report:

I. Summary of national needs identified by the research programs reviewed.
   A. On the basis of the best available evidence, place those needs in the context of the overall estimated potential work-related disease and injury burden.
   B. Discuss the choices made and alternatives that might be the focus of current or future attention.
   C. Comment on programs not selected by NIOSH for evaluation by the National Academies.

II. Assessment of how well the program goals.
   A. Were matched to the research program needs.
   B. Were adjusted to new information and inputs as the field of interest changed or program results became available.
III. Assessment of NIOSH overall performance in the research programs reviewed.
   A. Distribution of available inputs.
   B. Activities and outputs.
   C. Intermediate outcomes.
   D. Summary assessment of significant differences among the programs
   E. International impact.
   F. Leveraging of the NIOSH research activity with respect to other public and private research programs.
   G. Assessment of relative importance of external factors in permitting or preventing intermediate or end outcomes; attention paid to accounting for and planning within the constraints of external factors (not simply assigning lack of progress to external factors).
IV. Overall assessment of NIOSH impact on progress in reducing occupational injury and illness.
   A. Breakthrough knowledge.
   B. International impact.
   C. Addressing disparities.
   D. Targeting residual risks and intractable risks.
   E. Coordinating NIOSH research activity with respect to other public and private research programs.
   F. Impact on occupational safety and health.
V. Summary, Conclusions, and Recommendations.

B

Methods Section: Committee Information Gathering

This appendix provides additional detail regarding the methods used by the Institute of Medicine (IOM) Committee to Review the NIOSH Hearing Loss Research Program to gather information to carry out its work. These methods included reviewing written information from NIOSH, conducting site visits to facilities operated or used by NIOSH, inviting comments from stakeholders, and hearing presentations at two information-gathering meetings.

INFORMATION GATHERING

Written Information from NIOSH

The NIOSH Hearing Loss Research Program provided a roughly 400-page notebook of information to the committee in advance of the committee's first meeting. The notebook, referred to by NIOSH and the committee as the "evidence package," contained information on the history of the Hearing Loss Research Program; the program's resources, goals, and objectives; intramural research activities; extramural research funded by NIOSH; program products and technology transfer; and relevant NIOSH-wide processes and activities. The Hearing Loss Research Program and others in NIOSH provided extensive additional information to the committee in response to questions that arose during the evaluation process. All interactions and follow-up with NIOSH were carried out through

APPENDIX B

staff. A list of materials provided to the committee by NIOSH is found in Appendix C. In addition to written materials provided by NIOSH, the committee also had independent access to other NIOSH papers and conference materials.

Site Visits

In response to an invitation from NIOSH and after careful consideration, a subset of the committee made site visits to the Pittsburgh Research Laboratory on March 21, 2006, and to the Robert Taft Research Laboratory in Cincinnati, Ohio, on March 22, 2006. Committee members used the site visits to address specific questions that had arisen in the course of their review and to further inform their impressions from the materials provided by NIOSH. During the site visits, NIOSH staff provided committee members with tours of the research facilities and showed them the testing equipment available onsite. In Cincinnati, committee visitors also had the opportunity to visit the laboratory at the University of Cincinnati, where noise emissions from powered hand tools have been measured under a contract from the NIOSH Hearing Loss Research Program. Agendas for the site visits are presented in Box B-1.

Opportunity for Stakeholders to Comment on the NIOSH Hearing Loss Research Program

The committee was directed by the Framework Document to consider stakeholder input in assessing the impact and relevance of the NIOSH Hearing Loss Research Program. Issues of interest included whether stakeholder input was taken into consideration in shaping the NIOSH research program and stakeholders' views on the program's research activities and products.

The Framework Document did not specify the means for eliciting input from stakeholders. The committee determined that conducting a systematic survey was not feasible within the constraints of the project. As an alternative, the committee invited stakeholders to provide comments relevant to its evaluation of the impact and relevance of the NIOSH Hearing Loss Research Program. The objective was to assemble comments from a diverse group of organizations and individuals. Individual invitations to comment were sent to approximately 200 people and organizations. The invitation was also posted on a publicly available website.

Identification of Stakeholders

The committee identified possible stakeholders for the NIOSH Hearing Loss Research Program through several means. The research program provided a list of

**BOX B-1
Agendas for Site Visits**

**NIOSH Pittsburgh Research Laboratory
March 21, 2006**

9:30–11:00 a.m.	Pick up from airport	Ed Thimons, Branch Chief, Respiratory Hazard Control Branch (RHCB)
11:00–11:05 a.m.	Dr. Güner Gürtunca, Ph.D. Laboratory Director, Pittsburgh Research Laboratory	Bldg. 155, Conference Room
11:05–11:10 a.m.	R. J. Matetic, Branch Chief, Hearing Loss Prevention Branch (HLPB) • Introduction to Hearing Loss Program	
11:10–11:25 a.m.	Dr. Eric Bauer, Ph.D., P.E., Mining Engineer • Exposure Source and Dose	Bldg. 155, Conference Room

Engineering Controls 1

11:25–11:35 a.m.	Peter Kovalchik, Team Leader, Noise Control Team • Overview of Noise Control	Bldg. 154, Acoustical Testing Laboratory
11:35–12:25 p.m.	J. Shawn Peterson, Electrical Engineer • Coated Flight Bars—Continuous Mining Machine • Reverberation Chamber • Accreditation of Laboratory Facilities • Mist System—Roof Bolting Machine	
12:35–1:20 p.m.	Lunch and Worker Empowerment and Education Robert Randolph, Team Leader, Audiology and Intervention and Support Teams	Bldg. 155, Conference Room

Engineering Controls 2

1:20–1:50 p.m.	David Yantek, Mechanical Engineer • Hemi-anechoic Chamber • Shaker on Continuous Mining Machine Tail Section	Bldg. 153, Hemi-anechoic Chamber

APPENDIX B

1:50–2:05 p.m.	Adam Smith, Mechanical Engineer • Sound Intensity on Tail Roller—Continuous Mining Machine	
2:05–2:15 p.m.	David Yantek, Mechanical Engineer • Beam Forming Technique	
2:15–2:20 p.m.	Ellsworth Spencer, Mining Engineer • Longwall Pilot Study	
2:20–2:40 p.m.	Dr. Efrem Reeves, Ph.D., Acoustical Engineer • Communication and Personal Protective Equipment	Bldg. 154, Auditory Research Laboratory
2:40–3:00 p.m.	R. J. Matetic, BC, HLPB, and Ed Thimons, BC, RHCB • Mine Roof Simulator; Human Performance Research Mine; Full-Scale Continuous Miner Dust Gallery; Full-Scale Longwall Dust Gallery	
3:00 p.m.	Return to Airport	

NIOSH Cincinnati
Division of Applied Research and Technology (DART)
March 22, 2006

8:00 a.m.	Meet at Mariemont Inn • Drive to NIOSH Taft Laboratory • Building check-in with security	Greg Lotz, Ph.D. Assistant Director for Science (ADS), DART
8:30–9:00 a.m.	DART Conference Room, Taft Room 349 • Welcome and introductions • Plans for the day	Mary Lynn Woebkenberg, Ph.D., Director, DART Greg Lotz, ADS, DART
9:00–10:00 a.m.	Hearing Loss Research Program Labs, Taft 3rd Floor • Tour of Hearing Protector Lab and discussion of research • Tour of Audiometric Lab and discussion of research	William Murphy, Ph.D., DART
10:00–10:30 a.m.	Travel to University of Cincinnati	Charles Hayden, DART

continued

BOX B-1 Continued

10:30–11:15 a.m.	University of Cincinnati (UC), College of Engineering • Tour of UC/NIOSH Anechoic Lab	Charles Hayden, DART Jay Kim, Ph.D., Associate Professor, UC College of Engineering Ed Zechmann, DART
11:15–12:30 p.m.	Conference room (ERC 435, UC) • Discussion of NIOSH powered hand tools research; Q&A session	Charles Hayden, DART Jay Kim, Ph.D., Associate Professor, UC College of Engineering Ed Zechmann, DART
12:30–2:00 p.m.	Working lunch	
2:00–2:30 p.m.	Wrap-up discussion	Greg Lotz William Murphy Charles Hayden
2:30 p.m.	Return to airport	

its stakeholders, which included collaborators and partners. Working independently and drawing on suggestions from committee members and staff research, the committee identified as possible stakeholders individuals and organizations with an interest in audiology, hearing conservation, hearing protection devices, noise control engineering, and occupational epidemiologic research. This group included researchers from academia and private organizations, professional societies, organizations representing labor and industry, and others who deal directly with occupational hearing loss or were considered likely to be aware of this issue. Stakeholders were identified in a variety of industrial sectors, including construction, mining, agriculture, manufacturing, transportation, and the military. The committee also identified potential stakeholders among minority professional organizations and small business associations. The list of stakeholders included representatives of federal and state agencies as well as researchers and organizations in other countries.

APPENDIX B

Letters to Stakeholders

The invitation to comment on the NIOSH Hearing Loss Research Program was issued in a letter from committee chair Dr. Bernard Goldstein (see Box B-2). The committee staff sent the letter by e-mail in late January 2006 to each of the identified stakeholders. Committee members did not contact any stakeholders directly. The letter was also made available publicly from late-January through mid-May 2006 in a posting on a National Academies website. In addition, a NIOSH web page noted the opportunity for NIOSH stakeholders to provide input to the review and provided a link to the National Academies site. Interested stakeholders were asked to send their comments to the study staff via postal mail, e-mail, or the project website. Responses could be submitted anonymously through the website. The committee invited stakeholder comments on several points: familiarity with NIOSH activities and products related to occupational hearing loss and noise control; experience working with NIOSH; the relevance and impact of NIOSH's work over the past decade in occupational hearing loss and noise control; and the major research challenges over the past decade and significant emerging research needs in occupational hearing loss and noise control.

By June 2006, approximately 40 responses had been received. Stakeholder comments are available to the public through the National Academies Public Access file and were provided to NIOSH in their original form.

Overall, the NIOSH stakeholders who responded provided positive feedback. The committee recognizes that the responses to the request for comment are not necessarily representative of all NIOSH stakeholders. However, the comments provided to the committee gave helpful insights on responders' perspectives toward the NIOSH Hearing Loss Program and informed the committee's understanding of the program's relationship with some of its stakeholders.

Stakeholder Comments on Emerging Research Needs or Opportunities

To assist the committee in reviewing stakeholder input, the staff compiled the comments on significant emerging research needs or opportunities. This compilation is presented in Box B-3, with some comments captured in abbreviated form and others listed nearly verbatim. No attempt was made to evaluate the merits of individual stakeholder suggestions or to prioritize within or across the broad research categories used by the staff to group the comments. The presentation of these suggestions in the report does not represent an endorsement by the committee.

BOX B-2
Letter Inviting Comment on the NIOSH Hearing Loss Research Program

Dear Colleague:

I write as chair of the Institute of Medicine (IOM) Committee to Review the NIOSH Hearing Loss Research Program to invite your assistance in the work of this group. The committee's charge is derived from a request by the National Institute for Occupational Safety and Health (NIOSH) that the National Research Council and the Institute of Medicine convene individual committees to review as many as 15 NIOSH programs with respect to the impact and relevance of their work in reducing workplace injury and illness and to identify future directions their work might take. As part of our effort, we are seeking input and advice from a variety of individuals and organizations that we believe are likely to have an interest in occupational hearing loss and noise control.

The committee's charge is to examine the following issues for the NIOSH Hearing Loss Research Program:

(1) Progress in reducing workplace illness and injuries through occupational safety and health research, assessed on the basis of an analysis of relevant data about workplace illnesses and injuries and an evaluation of the effect that NIOSH research has had in reducing illness and injuries.

(2) Progress in targeting new research to the areas of occupational safety and health most relevant to future improvements in workplace protection.

(3) Significant emerging research areas that appear especially important in terms of their relevance to the mission of NIOSH.

The committee will evaluate the Hearing Loss Research Program using an assessment framework developed by the NRC/IOM Committee to Review the NIOSH Research Programs. The evaluation will consider what the NIOSH program is producing as well as whether the program can reasonably be credited with changes in workplace practices, or whether such changes are the result of other factors unrelated to NIOSH. For cases where impact is difficult to measure directly, the committee reviewing the Hearing Loss Research Program may use information on intermediate outcomes to evaluate performance.

NIOSH has provided information to the committee on its work on occupational hearing loss using four categories of research and research transfer activities: (1) development, implementation, and evaluation of effective hearing loss prevention programs; (2) evaluation of hearing protection devices; (3) development and use of engineering controls to reduce noise exposure; and (4) improved understanding of occupational hearing loss through surveillance and investigation of risk factors.

We would be very grateful for your comments on any of several points. It would be valuable for the committee to know whether you are familiar with NIOSH activities and products related to occupational hearing loss and noise control and what kind of experience you may have had working with the agency or its products. The committee would be particularly interested in comments you may have on the relevance and impact of NIOSH's work on occupational hearing loss and noise control over the past 10 years in any of the four areas of research it has defined.

In addition, we would value your views on two other matters included in the committee's charge. First, what do you see as having been the major research needs and challenges over the past 10 years in occupational hearing loss and noise control? Second, what do you see as significant emerging research needs or opportunities concerning occupational hearing loss and noise control?

The committee will review the comments it receives at its two remaining meetings, which will be held on February 23–24 and March 30–31, 2006. We encourage you to submit your comments in time for consideration at the February meeting, if possible. You are welcome to comment as an interested individual or from the perspective of your organization. In addition, you should feel free to share this letter with other individuals or organizations with an interest in occupational hearing loss.

If you wish to comment, please do so through our IOM staff, using any of a variety of routes: e-mail, mail, fax, telephone, or through the project website (where providing name and affiliation is optional). Contact details are provided at the end of this letter. Please note that any written comments submitted to the committee (whether by mail, e-mail, fax, or the project website) will be included in the study's public access file. If you have any questions about contacting the committee or providing materials for the committee's consideration, I encourage you to speak with our study director Lois Joellenbeck or her colleague Jane Durch.

Thank you very much for any assistance you can provide to our study committee as we conduct our review of the NIOSH Hearing Loss Research Program.

       Sincerely,

       Bernard Goldstein, M.D.
       Chair, Committee to Review the NIOSH Hearing Loss
       Research Program

Submitting Comments to the Study Committee

Mail:
 Dr. Lois Joellenbeck
 Institute of Medicine, Keck 775
 500 Fifth Street, N.W.
 Washington, DC 20001

BOX B-3
Emerging Research Areas in Occupational Hearing Loss and Noise Control Suggested by Stakeholders

Hearing Loss Prevention Programs (HLPPs)
Overcoming barriers to hearing conservation programs
Best practices for implementing hearing conservation programs and hearing loss prevention training
Evaluation of the effectiveness of hearing conservation programs and detection of significant threshold shifts
Methods of motivating and training employees in hearing conservation
Documentation of the benefits of HLPPs, over and above the prevention of noise-induced hearing loss
Practical limits of hearing conservation programs that rely on use of hearing protection devices
Development of methods and technologies to increase the use of hearing protection by miners as a component of a hearing conservation program

Hearing Evaluations
Analysis of the forced-whisper test
Markers for early threshold shift
Early indicators of hearing loss
Evaluating the most appropriate audiometric test frequencies for monitoring noise-induced hearing loss
Assessment of audiograms to determine if noise-induced hearing loss was a causative factor in the audiometric profile
Monitoring hearing more frequently in nonclinical settings

Hearing Protection Devices (HPDs)
Developing more reliable and cost-effective hearing protection and hearing testing equipment
Reasons for HPD failure in the real world
Improved mechanisms for HPD evaluation
Determination of reasons for the discrepancy between field and laboratory attenuation evaluations
Evaluation of HPD performance in individual users
Development and dissemination of HPDs with better sound quality and targeted attenuation; their benefits and limitations
Developing HPDs that maintain situational awareness and enhance communication-in-noise
Effective applications of "augmented" HPDs
Performance of level-dependent and electronic hearing protectors
Effective methods of motivating workers to wear HPDs correctly
Improved and validated real-world assessments of the performance of hearing protection in the workplace
Relationship between HPDs, hearing loss, and occupational injuries
NIOSH should support American National Standards Institute (ANSI) in the development and particularly the dissemination of hearing protector standards
Labeling of hearing protectors
Determining the actual incentives that will change worker behavior to use hearing protection

Noise Metrics
Developing "kurtosis" as a noise metric
Noise exposure measurement and estimation techniques

Impulsive Noise
The effects of impulse or impact noise
Measurement of impact noise
Develop damage risk criteria for impulse noise and blast, and intervention or mitigation of acute acoustic trauma

Noise Control
Working with the industry to reduce noise levels
Further research and publication of noise control approaches
Improved devices for noise control
Targeting general categories of sources is impractical. Instead, NIOSH should support development of noise control and acoustical engineering curricula at the undergraduate level to make plant engineers more aware of issues and solutions
Development and application of ambient noise cancellation technology
Organizational factors in lack of compliance with noise exposure limits (lack of feasible engineering controls, not using feasible controls, etc.)
Validation of engineering noise control research products with in-mine tests under actual mining conditions for full shifts with quantification of the reduction in miners' noise exposure
Research to assist MSHA in moving promising engineering and administrative noise controls to the technologically achievable category
Reducing noise levels associated with air arcing
Developing cost-effective engineering controls that can be integrated into industry process and procedures
Determining how existing engineering controls can be augmented to further reduce the potential for hearing loss

Product Design
Design more technology to reduce cab noise
Improve in-cab warning signal design
Product noise labeling
Overcoming obstacles to communication in noisy environments

Information for Industry and Workers
More information on noise emissions, noise control measures, and noise abatement approaches in user-friendly format
Collection of training materials
Collection of testimonials by recognized people and the average worker, voicing their perceived consequences of failed personal protection
Effective training materials relevant to young, inexperienced miners
Continued growth in mining and construction research

continued

BOX B-3 Continued

Surveillance
Ongoing research to monitor and assess the magnitude of occupational noise-induced hearing loss among miners

Evidence Base for Regulation and Prevention Programs
Translational research to produce and disseminate evidence-based interventions
Evidence-based input for regulatory requirements

Biological Factors
Determining the genetic, life-style, and dietary factors in humans that may underlie the well-known intersubject variability in noise-induced hearing loss (need for correlation studies)
Methods for separating age and other factors contributing to hearing loss
Hearing loss susceptibility in children

Prevention and Treatment
Pharmacologic intervention for prevention and remediation of noise trauma
Mechanisms of hair cell death and the possible benefits of otoprotectants

Other Contributors to Hearing Loss
More knowledge and research into determining which chemicals affect hearing
Effects of personal listening devices on hearing

High-Risk Groups or Vulnerable Populations
Effects of noise on aging workers
Interventions to promote hearing health in a diverse workforce
Dealing with hearing-impaired workers in the workplace and the potential use of hearing aids or hearing protection for such employees
Hearing loss prevention programs for underserved worker populations, such as the lawn care industry, the car wash industry, and musicians
Noise and hearing impairment as risk factors for injury among construction workers
Research to identify and assess ototoxic hazards for miners

Nonauditory Effects of Noise
Effect of noise exposure on blood pressure
Research to identify and assess nonauditory health effects of noise on miners

Appendix B

Stakeholder Respondents

The following individuals responded to the committee's invitation for comments on the NIOSH Hearing Loss Research Program:

Marin Allen
National Institutes of Health

Elliott Berger
E·A·R/Aearo Company

David Bies
Adelaide University

Jay Buckey
Dartmouth-Hitchcock Medical Center

Kathryn Butcher
National Ground Water Association

Kathleen Campbell
Southern Illinois University School of Medicine

Brent Chamberlain
Queenstake Resources USA Inc.

COL David Chandler
U.S. Army

William Daniell
University of Washington

Diane S. DeGaetano
Merial

Kyle Dennis
Department of Veterans Affairs

Robert Dobie
University of California, Davis

Albert G. Duble
Member, Institute of Noise Control Engineering (INCE)

Ronald W. Edgell
Silver Bell Mining

John Erdreich
Ostergaard Acoustical Associates

Laurence Fechter
Veterans Affairs Loma Linda Healthcare System

Jeffrey Goldberg
Custom Protect Ear, Inc.

Lee Hager
Sonomax Hearing Healthcare

Donald Henderson
State University of New York at Buffalo

Lonny Hofer
(No affiliation provided)

Ann-Christin Johnson
Karolinska Institute

Madeleine Kerr
University of Minnesota

Robert Kline-Schoder
Creare Incorporated

Joseph LaMonica
Bituminous Coal Operators' Association

Eric LePage
OAEricle Laboratory

Peter McAllister
Adelaide University

Brian Metcalf
(No affiliation provided)

Luc Mongeau
Purdue University

Rick Neitzel
University of Washington

Richard J. Peppin
Scantek, Inc.

Susan Randolph
American Association of Occupational Health Nurses

CDR Glen Rovig
U.S. Navy

Emmett Russell
International Union of Operating Engineers

Scott Schneider
Laborers' Health and Safety Fund of North America

Paul Schomer
Acoustical Society of America

Kathy Sotkovski
(No affiliation provided)

Martin Walker
Federal Motor Carrier Safety Administration

Laurie Wells
National Hearing Conservation Association

William Yost
Parmly Hearing Institute, Loyola University Chicago

APPENDIX B

COMMITTEE MEETINGS

The committee held three face-to-face meetings during the course of this study. The first two meetings included open sessions for information gathering. The agendas for these open sessions appear below. The third meeting was held in closed session. After the third meeting, the committee held four conference calls in order to finalize the report.

Meeting I
January 5–6, 2006
The Keck Center of the National Academies
500 Fifth Street, N.W.
Washington, D.C.

Thursday, January 5, 2006

10:15 a.m.	Introductory remarks *Bernard Goldstein, M.D.* *Chair, Committee to Review the NIOSH Hearing Loss Research Program* Introductions by committee members and meeting attendees
10:30	Study Context and Goals, Sponsor Perspective *Lewis Wade, Ph.D.* *Senior Science Advisor, NIOSH* Discussion
11:00	Evaluation Framework *David H. Wegman, M.D., M.Sc.* *Chair, Committee on the Review of NIOSH Research Programs* Discussion
Noon	Lunch
1:00 p.m.	Overview of the NIOSH Hearing Loss Research Program *W. Gregory Lotz, Ph.D.* *Associate Director for Science* *Division of Applied Research and Technology, NIOSH*

Discussion

1:50 NIOSH Hearing Loss Research Program: Research Goal 1:
Contribute to the development, implementation, and
evaluation of effective hearing loss prevention programs
Carol M. Stephenson, Ph.D.
Chief, Training Research and Evaluation Branch,
Education and Information Division, NIOSH

Discussion

2:30 NIOSH Hearing Loss Research Program: Research Goal 2:
Reduce hearing loss through interventions targeting personal
protective equipment
William J. Murphy, Ph.D.
Co-Team Leader, Hearing Loss Prevention Team
Division of Applied Research and Technology, NIOSH

Discussion

3:10 Break

3:25 NIOSH Hearing Loss Research Program: Research Goal 3:
Develop engineering controls to reduce noise exposures
R. J. Matetic, M.S.
Chief, Hearing Loss Prevention Branch
Pittsburgh Research Laboratory, NIOSH

Discussion

4:05 NIOSH Hearing Loss Research Program: Research Goal 4:
Contribute to reductions in hearing loss through the
understanding of causative mechanisms
Rickie R. Davis, Ph.D.
Co-Team Leader, Hearing Loss Prevention Team
Division of Applied Research and Technology, NIOSH

Discussion

4:45 Adjourn Open Session

Friday, January 6, 2006

9:30 a.m.   Discussion with NIOSH on study task and Hearing Loss Research Program, as needed

11:00   Adjourn Open Session

**Meeting II
February 23–24, 2006
The Keck Center of the National Academies
500 Fifth Street, N.W.
Washington, D.C.**

Thursday, February 23, 2006

11:00 a.m.   Introductory remarks
Bernard Goldstein, M.D.
Chair, Committee to Review the NIOSH Hearing Loss Research Program

Introductions by committee members and meeting attendees

11:15   Questions and discussion with NIOSH representatives

12:15 p.m.   Lunch

1:00   Presentations by selected NIOSH stakeholders

Noah Sexias, Ph.D.
Professor of Environmental and Occupational Health Sciences
University of Washington

Discussion

1:40   Mine Safety and Health Administration (MSHA)

John Seiler, P.E.
Chief, Physical and Toxic Agents Division
Directorate of Technical Support, MSHA

Melinda Pon
Special Assistant to the Administrator for Coal Mine Safety and Health, MSHA

Discussion

2:20 Occupational Safety and Health Administration (OSHA)

Jim Maddux
Director, Office of Maritime Standards and Guidance
OSHA

Mike Seymour
Acting Deputy Director, Office of Maritime Standards and Guidance
OSHA

Discussion

3:00 Environmental Protection Agency (EPA)

Ken Feith
Senior Scientist/Advisor
Office of Air and Radiation, EPA
    (by telephone)

Discussion

3:45 Additional discussion among presenters, NIOSH, committee

4:45 Adjourn open session

ACKNOWLEDGMENTS

The committee would like to extend its sincere gratitude to the NIOSH staff. The Hearing Loss Research Program staff at both the Pittsburgh Research Laboratory and the Robert Taft Laboratory in Cincinnati faced the substantial task of assembling the initial set of materials that were provided to the committee for this study. They also assembled a considerable amount of material in response to the

APPENDIX B

committee's requests for additional information and devoted time and effort to ensure the success of the committee's site visits. The committee extends particular thanks to the NIOSH staff who gave presentations or responded to questions from the committee at its meetings or site visits, including Dr. Eric Bauer, Dr. Rickie Davis, Dr. Güner Gürtunca, Mr. Charles Hayden II, Dr. Peter Kovalchik, Dr. W. Gregory Lotz, Dr. R.J. Matetic, Dr. Thais Morata, Dr. William Murphy, Mr. J. Shawn Peterson, Mr. Robert Randolph, Dr. Efrem Reeves, Mr. Adam Smith, Mr. Ellsworth Spencer, Dr. Carol Stephenson, Dr. Mark Stephenson, Mr. Ed Thimons, Dr. Lewis Wade, Dr. Mary Lynn Woebkenberg, and Mr. David Yantek. The committee also thanks NIOSH staff member Mr. Rohit Verma, Dr. Jay Kim of the University of Cincinnati, and Mr. Edward Zechmann of Constella.

The committee thanks as well the many members of the communities involved in occupational hearing loss prevention outside NIOSH who contributed to the study by providing comments on the NIOSH Hearing Loss Research Program, making presentations at the committee's meetings, or providing additional information in response to committee requests. In addition to the individuals listed earlier in this appendix, the committee wants to acknowledge Mr. Mark Rotariu of the National Institute on Deafness and Other Communication Disorders; Mr. Ryan German, Ms. Shelly McCoy, Mr. Gregory Meikle, Ms. Melinda Pon, and Mr. John Seiler of MSHA; Mr. Ken Feith and Ms. Catrice Jefferson of EPA; Mr. Jim Maddux and Mr. Mike Seymour of OSHA; Dr. Noah Seixas of the University of Washington; and Dr. David Wegman of the University of Massachusetts Lowell and chair of the National Academies Committee for the Review of NIOSH Research Programs.

The committee would especially like to recognize the assistance of Dr. W. Gregory Lotz. Dr. Lotz served as the committee's point of contact for the NIOSH Hearing Loss Research Program and was tireless and gracious in his efforts to respond to the committee's many information requests and questions. The committee is also grateful for the assistance of Dr. Raymond Sinclair, who ably and patiently acted as a liaison between the committee and NIOSH as a whole.

The committee appreciates the support of Andrew Pope, director of the IOM Board on Health Sciences Policy, and Evan Douple and Sammantha Magsino, who serve as staff to the Committee for the Review of NIOSH Research Program. In addition, several members of the National Academies staff helped in the report review, preproduction, dissemination, and financial management for the report, including Judy Estep, Amy Haas, Clyde Behney, Bronwyn Schrecker, Elisabeth Reese, Tyjen Tsai, Sally Stanfield, Hallie Wilfert, Christine Stencel, David Codrea, and Cathie Berkley.

C

Information Provided by the NIOSH Hearing Loss Research Program

Some of these materials are available online at the following NIOSH website: *http://www.cdc.gov/niosh/nas/hlr/*. All of the materials are available for review at the National Academies through the study's public access file.

AAA (American Academy of Audiology). 2003. Position Statement: Preventing Noise-Induced Occupational Hearing Loss. Reston, VA: AAA.

Achutan C, Tubbs RL, Habes DJ. 2004. NIOSH Health Hazard Evaluation Report, HETA 2004-0014-2929: Navajo Agricultural Products Industry, Farmington, New Mexico. Cincinnati, OH: NIOSH.

ANSI (American National Standards Institute). 1992. ANSI S12.15-1992 (ASA 106-1992). *For Acoustics—Portable Electric Power Tools, Stationary and Fixed Electric Power Tools, and Gardening Appliances—Measurement of Sound Emitted.* New York: Acoustical Society of America. Annotated.

Davis R. 2006. Research Goal 4: Contribute to Reductions in Hearing Loss Through the Understanding of Causative Mechanisms. Presentation to the Committee to Review the NIOSH Hearing Loss Research Program, Meeting I, January 5. Washington, DC.

Davis RR, Murphy WJ, Byrne DC, Franks JR. 2006. Comfort and Personal NRR in a Longitudinal Study of Highly Experienced Earplug Users (slide set). Presentation for NHCA Conference, Tampa, FL, February 17–19.

Franks JR. 1996. Analysis of Audiograms for a Large Cohort of Noise-Exposed Miners. Unpublished technical report. Cincinnati, OH: NIOSH.

Franks JR. 1997. Initial Results from Analysis of Audiograms for Non-Coal Miners. Cincinnati, OH: NIOSH. Memorandum. June 16.

Franks JR. 1997. Prevalence of Hearing Loss for Noise-Exposed Metal/Nonmetal Miners. Unpublished technical report. Cincinnati, OH: NIOSH.

Harney JM, King BF, Tubbs RL, Hayden CS, Kardous CA, Khan A, Mickelsen RL, Wilson RD. 2005. NIOSH Health Hazard Evaluation Report, HETA 2000-0191-2960: Immigration and Naturalization Service, National Firearms Unit, Altoona, Pennsylvania. Cincinnati, OH: NIOSH.

Hodgson M, Li D. 2004. Active Control of Workplace Noise Exposure. Final report prepared for the National Institute for Occupational Safety and Health under Grant No. 1 R01 OH003963-01A1. University of British Columbia. October.

ISO (International Organization for Standardization). No date. Procedures for general qualification for anechoic and hemi-anechoic rooms. In: ISO 3745. *Acoustics—Determination of Sound Power Levels of Noise Sources Using Sound Pressure—Precision Methods for Anechoic and Hemi-Anechoic Rooms.* Geneva, Switzerland: ISO. Annex A. Annotated.

ISO. 1994. ISO 3744, 2nd ed. 1994-05-01. *Acoustics—Determination of Sound Power Levels of Noise Sources Using Sound Pressure—Engineering Method in an Essentially Free Field over a Reflecting Plane.* Geneva, Switzerland: ISO. Annotated.

JGS Consulting. No date. Preliminary Calculations for NIOSH Cincinnati–University of Cincinnati Anechoic Chamber (Excel file). Austin, TX: JGS Consulting.

JGS Consulting. 2001. Engineering Report: Evaluation of the Adequacy of the Anechoic Chamber at the University of Cincinnati for the Measurement and Reporting of Noise Emissions from Power Tools and Equipment. Order No. 0000136449. Austin, TX: JGS Consulting.

Joseph AR, Punch JL, Stephenson MR, Murphy WJ. 2006. The Sound Attenuation Fit Estimator. Poster for NHCA Conference, Tampa, FL, February 17–19.

Joseph A, Punch J, Stephenson M, Murphy B, Paneth N, Wolfe E. 2006. The Effects of Training Modality on Earplug Performance (slide set). Presentation for NHCA Conference, Tampa, FL, February 17–19.

Kovalchik P, Johnson M, Burdisso R, Duda F, Durr M. 2002. A Noise Control for Continuous Miners. Paper for presentation at the 10th International Meeting on Low Frequency Noise and Vibration and Its Control, York, England, September 11–13.

Lotz WG. 2005. An Overview of the Hearing Loss Research Program at NIOSH. Presentation slides (May 5). Cincinnati, OH: NIOSH.

Lotz WG. 2005. An Overview of the Hearing Loss Research Program at NIOSH (Note Pages). Cincinnati, OH: NIOSH.

Lotz WG (NIOSH). 2005. FW: your message on my voicemail. E-mail to L Joellenbeck, Institute of Medicine. November 1.

Lotz WG (NIOSH). 2005. RE: follow-up on yesterday's call. E-mail to J Durch and L Joellenbeck, Institute of Medicine. November 30.

Lotz WG (NIOSH). 2005. FW: Draft agenda for January 5-6 meeting. E-mail to L Joellenbeck, Institute of Medicine. December 13.

Lotz WG (NIOSH). 2006. Overview of NIOSH Hearing Loss Research Program. Presentation to the Committee to Review the NIOSH Hearing Loss Research Program, Meeting I, January 5. Washington, DC.

Lotz WG (NIOSH). 2006. FW: NIOSH HLR Program Stakeholders List. E-mail to L Joellenbeck, Institute of Medicine. January 17.

Lotz WG (NIOSH). 2006. FW: request for info. E-mail to L Joellenbeck, Institute of Medicine. January 20.

Lotz WG (NIOSH). 2006. FW: NIOSH eNews Flash—Invitation to NORA Symposium 2006. E-mail to L Joellenbeck, Institute of Medicine. January 20.

Lotz WG (NIOSH). 2006. An additional contact for the stakeholder list. E-mail to L Joellenbeck, Institute of Medicine. January 22.

Lotz WG (NIOSH). 2006. FW: updated request list. E-mail to L Joellenbeck, Institute of Medicine. January 23.

Lotz WG (NIOSH). 2006. NIOSH HLRP Org. Chart. E-mail to L Joellenbeck, Institute of Medicine. January 30.

Lotz WG (NIOSH). 2006. 2001 NORA HLRP Proposal. E-mail to L Joellenbeck, Institute of Medicine. January 30.

Lotz WG (NIOSH). 2006. FW: request for info—NOES. E-mail to L Joellenbeck, Institute of Medicine. January 30.

Lotz WG (NIOSH). 2006. RE: additional info and document requests. E-mail to L Joellenbeck, Institute of Medicine. January 30.

Lotz WG (NIOSH). 2006. FW: NIOSH HLRP Contracts and CRADAs. E-mail to L Joellenbeck, Institute of Medicine. January 31.

Lotz WG (NIOSH). 2006. RE: NIOSH HLRP Extramural Projects. E-mail to L Joellenbeck, Institute of Medicine. February 1.

Lotz WG (NIOSH). 2006. RE: NIOSH HLR Program website. E-mail to L Joellenbeck, Institute of Medicine. February 2.

Lotz WG (NIOSH). 2006. Re: NIOSH HLRP Extramural Projects #2. E-mail to L Joellenbeck, Institute of Medicine. February 7.

Lotz WG (NIOSH). 2006. BLS data from OSHA 300 log. E-mail to L Joellenbeck, Institute of Medicine. February 16.

APPENDIX C

Lotz WG (NIOSH). 2006. FW: BLS data from OSHA 300 log. E-mail to L Joellenbeck, Institute of Medicine. February 17.

Lotz WG (NIOSH). 2006. RE: document and detail requests—responses 1 and 2 part 1. E-mail to L Joellenbeck, Institute of Medicine. February 20.

Lotz WG (NIOSH). 2006. FW: NIOSH Peer Review Summary. E-mail to L Joellenbeck, Institute of Medicine. February 22.

Lotz WG (NIOSH). 2006. EarTalk follow-up. E-mail to L Joellenbeck, Institute of Medicine. March 17.

Lotz WG (NIOSH). 2006. Field Verification of HPD Attenuation. E-mail to L Joellenbeck, Institute of Medicine. March 17.

Lotz WG (NIOSH). 2006. FW: NIOSH presentations to NHCA. E-mail to L Joellenbeck, Institute of Medicine. March 17.

Lotz WG (NIOSH). 2006. RE: some follow-up questions on RG 2 and 4. E-mail to L Joellenbeck, Institute of Medicine. March 17.

Lotz WG (NIOSH). 2006. FW: additional information request. E-mail to L Joellenbeck, Institute of Medicine. March 18.

Lotz WG (NIOSH). 2006. FW: NIOSH presentations to NHCA. E-mail to L Joellenbeck, Institute of Medicine. March 18.

Lotz WG (NIOSH). 2006. FW: Schedule for NIOSH Cincinnati Site Visit. E-mail to L Joellenbeck, Institute of Medicine. March 18.

Lotz WG (NIOSH). 2006. FW: additional questions related to Research Goal 3. E-mail to L Joellenbeck, Institute of Medicine. March 20.

Lotz WG (2006). FW: Powered Hand Tools CRADA. E-mail to L Joellenbeck, Institute of Medicine. March 20.

Lotz WG (NIOSH). 2006. FW: RFA—Centers for Construction Safety and Health. E-mail to L Joellenbeck, Institute of Medicine. March 27.

Lotz WG (NIOSH). 2006. RE: two requests for info. E-mail to L Joellenbeck, Institute of Medicine. April 20.

Lotz WG (NIOSH). 2006. Re: two requests for info. E-mail to L Joellenbeck, Institute of Medicine. April 26.

Lotz WG (NIOSH). 2006. RE: info request. E-mail to L Joellenbeck, Institute of Medicine. May 26.

Lotz WG (NIOSH). 2006. RE: info request. E-mail to L Joellenbeck, Institute of Medicine. May 30.

Lotz WG (NIOSH). 2006. Paper on hearing loss in carpenters. E-mail to L Joellenbeck, Institute of Medicine. May 30.

Lotz WG (NIOSH). Re: update on timing, and question. E-mail to L Joellenbeck, Institute of Medicine. June 14.

Lotz WG (NIOSH). 2006. Re: seek technical review of figure and caption. E-mail to L Joellenbeck, Institute of Medicine. July 21.

Lotz WG (NIOSH). 2006. RE: seek technical review of figure and caption. E-mail to L Joellenbeck, Institute of Medicine. August 1.

Matetic RJ (NIOSH). 2006. Agenda—PRL Visit. E-mail to L Joellenbeck, Institute of Medicine. March 14.

Matetic RJ. 2006. Research Goal 3: Develop Engineering Controls to Reduce Noise Exposure. Presentation to the Committee to Review the NIOSH Hearing Loss Research Program, Meeting I, January 5. Washington, DC.

Morata TC. 2006. Best Practices, International Standards and Legislations Regarding Chemical Exposure in the Workplace and the Risk of Hearing Loss (slide set). Presentation for NHCA Conference, Tampa, FL, February 17–19.

Murphy WJ. 2006. Research Goal 2: Reducing Hearing Loss Through Interventions Targeting Personal Protective Equipment. Presentation to the Committee to Review the NIOSH Hearing Loss Research Program, Meeting I, January 5. Washington, DC.

National Safety Council and NIOSH. 2000. Listen up! Learn how to protect your hearing. *Today's Supervisor* 64(2):1–19.

National Safety Council and NIOSH. 2000. Sound advice—Protect your ears in noisy work environments. *Safeworker* 74(February):1–15.

NIOSH (National Institute for Occupational Safety and Health). No date. NIOSH Hearing Loss Publications. DHHS (NIOSH) Pub. No. 2001-102. Cincinnati, OH: NIOSH.

NIOSH. No date. NIOSH Work-Related Hearing Loss. DHHS (NIOSH) Pub. No. 2001-103. Cincinnati, OH: NIOSH.

NIOSH. 1988. A proposed national strategy for the prevention of noise-induced hearing loss. In: *Proposed National Strategies for the Prevention of Leading Work-Related Diseases and Injuries*, Part 2. Cincinnati, OH: NIOSH. Pp. 51–63.

NIOSH. 1996. *Preventing Occupational Hearing Loss—A Practical Guide.* DHHS (NIOSH) Pub. No. 96-110. Cincinnati, OH: NIOSH.

NIOSH. 1998. *Criteria for a Recommended Standard. Occupational Noise Exposure: Revised Criteria 1998.* DHHS (NIOSH) Pub. No. 98-126. Cincinnati, OH: NIOSH.

NIOSH. 1998. *Health Hazard Evaluations: Noise and Hearing Loss 1986–1997.* DHHS (NIOSH) Pub. No. 99-106. Cincinnati, OH: NIOSH.

NIOSH. 1998. *National Institute for Occupational Safety and Health Strategic Plan 1997–2002.* DHHS (NIOSH) Pub. No. 98-137. Washington, DC: U.S. Department of Health and Human Services.

NIOSH. 1998. White Paper: Engineering Noise Controls and Personal Protective Equipment. Paper prepared for Control of Workplace Hazards for the 21st Century: Setting the Research Agenda (conference and workshop), Chicago, March 10–12.

NIOSH. 1999. National Institute for Occupational Safety and Health; Safety and Health Interventions in the Construction Industry; Notice of Availability of Funds. (Program Announcement 99062). *Federal Register* 64(64):16468–164470.

NIOSH. 2000. NORA Proposals: NIOSH FY2001 Project Forms. Cincinnati, OH: NIOSH.

NIOSH. 2001. Agenda for Review Meeting: Identifying Effective Hearing Loss Prevention Strategies. Washington, DC, January 11.

NIOSH. 2001. Identifying Effective Hearing Loss Prevention Strategies (reviewers' comments). Washington, DC: NIOSH.

NIOSH. 2001. *Proceedings: Best Practices in Hearing Loss Prevention.* Detroit, Michigan. October 28, 1999. DHHS (NIOSH) Pub. No. 2001-157. Cincinnati, OH: NIOSH.

NIOSH. 2002. NIOSH Policy on External Peer Review of Intramural Projects. Cincinnati, OH: NIOSH.

NIOSH. 2003. Centers for Construction Safety and Health. RFA No. RFA-OH-04-002. Bethesda, MD: Department of Health and Human Services.

NIOSH. 2004. Customer Satisfaction Survey. NIOSH Publications and Information Services. In: Evidence for the National Academies' Committee to Review the NIOSH Hearing Loss Research Program. Cincinnati, OH: NIOSH. Appendix E.

NIOSH. 2004. *Worker Health Chartbook, 2004.* DHHS Pub No. 2004-146. Cincinnati, OH: NIOSH.

NIOSH. 2005. A Brief Description of the NIOSH Hearing Loss Research Program. Cincinnati, OH: NIOSH.

NIOSH. 2005. Collaborations of NIOSH Scientists with Extramural Scientists. Cincinnati, OH: NIOSH.

NIOSH. 2005. Cooperative Agreements: NIOSH Staff Involvement on Extramural Awards. Cincinnati, OH: NIOSH.

NIOSH. 2005. NIOSH FY 2006 PART Summary. Cincinnati, OH: NIOSH.

NIOSH. 2005. NIOSH FY2006 Project Form. Research Proposal Information Summary: Hearing Loss Prevention for Shipyard Workers. Cincinnati, OH: NIOSH.

NIOSH. 2005. NIOSH Hearing Loss Prevention Futures Workshop. Workshop announcement. Cincinnati, OH: NIOSH.

NIOSH. 2005. NIOSH Hearing Loss Prevention Program Logic Model. Cincinnati, OH: NIOSH.

NIOSH. 2005. NIOSH Policy on External Peer Review of Intramural Projects: Addendum—Peer Review Quality Gateway. Cincinnati, OH: NIOSH.

NIOSH. 2005. NIOSH Program Area Funding FY 1997–2004. Cincinnati, OH: NIOSH.

NIOSH. 2005. Introduction and Highlights. In: NIOSH Hearing Loss Research Program: Evidence for the National Academies' Committee to Review the NIOSH Hearing Loss Research Program. Cincinnati, OH: NIOSH. Pp. 1–5.

NIOSH. 2005. NIOSH Overview. In: NIOSH Hearing Loss Research Program: Evidence for the National Academies' Committee to Review the NIOSH Hearing Loss Research Program. Cincinnati, OH: NIOSH. Pp. 7–17.

NIOSH. 2005. NIOSH Hearing Loss Research Program: Overview. In: NIOSH Hearing Loss Research Program: Evidence for the National Academies' Committee to Review the NIOSH Hearing Loss Research Program. Cincinnati, OH: NIOSH. Pp. 19–40.

NIOSH. 2005. Research Goal 1: Contribute to the Development, Implementation, and Evaluation of Effective Hearing Loss Prevention Programs. In: NIOSH Hearing Loss Research Program: Evidence for the National Academies' Committee to Review the NIOSH Hearing Loss Research Program. Cincinnati, OH: NIOSH. Pp. 43–75.

NIOSH. 2005. Research Goal 2: Reduce Hearing Loss Through Interventions Targeting Personal Protective Equipment. In: NIOSH Hearing Loss Research Program: Evidence for the National Academies' Committee to Review the NIOSH Hearing Loss Research Program. Cincinnati, OH: NIOSH. Pp. 77–99.

NIOSH. 2005. Research Goal 3: Develop Engineering Controls to Reduce Noise Exposure. In: NIOSH Hearing Loss Research Program: Evidence for the National Academies' Committee to Review the NIOSH Hearing Loss Research Program. Cincinnati, OH: NIOSH. Pp. 101–123.

NIOSH. 2005. Research Goal 4: Contribute to Reductions in Hearing Loss Through the Understanding of Causative Mechanisms. In: NIOSH Hearing Loss Research Program: Evidence for the National Academies' Committee to Review the NIOSH Hearing Loss Research Program. Cincinnati, OH: NIOSH. Pp. 125–155.

NIOSH. 2005. Emerging Issues. In: NIOSH Hearing Loss Research Program: Evidence for the National Academies' Committee to Review the NIOSH Hearing Loss Research Program. Cincinnati, OH: NIOSH. Pp. 157–162.

NIOSH. 2005. Selected NIOSH Sponsored Workshops and Conferences Related to the HLR Program. In: NIOSH Hearing Loss Research Program: Evidence for the National Academies' Committee to Review the NIOSH Hearing Loss Research Program. Cincinnati, OH: NIOSH. Pp. 8A-1–8A-8.

NIOSH. 2005. Databases. In: NIOSH Hearing Loss Research Program: Evidence for the National Academies' Committee to Review the NIOSH Hearing Loss Research Program. Cincinnati, OH: NIOSH. Pp. 8B-1–8B-15.

NIOSH. 2005. Partnerships. In: NIOSH Hearing Loss Research Program: Evidence for the National Academies' Committee to Review the NIOSH Hearing Loss Research Program. Cincinnati, OH: NIOSH. Pp. 8C-1–8C-21.

NIOSH. 2005. Professional Staff. In: NIOSH Hearing Loss Research Program: Evidence for the National Academies' Committee to Review the NIOSH Hearing Loss Research Program. Cincinnati, OH: NIOSH. Pp. 9-1–9-50.

NIOSH. 2005. NIOSH Hearing Loss Research Program: The NIOSH Office of Health Communication. In: NIOSH Hearing Loss Research Program: Evidence for the National Academies' Committee to Review the NIOSH Hearing Loss Research Program. Cincinnati, OH: NIOSH. Appendix D.

NIOSH. 2005. NORA Hearing Loss Team Recommendations, 2005. In: NIOSH Hearing Loss Research Program: Evidence for the National Academies' Committee to Review the NIOSH Hearing Loss Research Program. Cincinnati, OH: NIOSH. Appendix H.

NIOSH. 2005. NIOSH Office of Extramural Programs Overview. In: NIOSH Hearing Loss Research Program: Evidence for the National Academies' Committee to Review the NIOSH Hearing Loss Research Program. Cincinnati, OH: NIOSH. Appendix I.

NIOSH. 2006. Hearing Loss Extramural Award Summary Through FY 2005. Cincinnati, OH: NIOSH.

NIOSH. 2006. Background on Funding for Mining Within the NIOSH Budget. Cincinnati, OH: NIOSH.

NIOSH. 2006. NA/IOM Hearing Loss Research Program Visit Itinerary—March 22, 2006 (NIOSH Cincinnati). Cincinnati, OH: NIOSH.

NIOSH. 2006. NAS Hearing Loss Visit Itinerary—March 21, 2006. Pittsburgh, PA: NIOSH.

NIOSH. 2006. National Institute for Occupational Safety and Health Organization Chart. Cincinnati, OH: NIOSH.

NIOSH. 2006. NIOSH Hearing Loss Research Program. Cincinnati, OH: NIOSH.

NIOSH. 2006. NIOSH Hearing Loss Research Program: 2005 Futures Workshop. Cincinnati, OH: NIOSH.

NIOSH. 2006. NIOSH Hearing Loss Research Program Budget FY97–FY05 (Excel spreadsheet). Cincinnati, OH: NIOSH.

NIOSH. 2006. NIOSH Hearing Loss Research Program: Contracts and CRADAs Supported by Intramural Projects. Cincinnati, OH: NIOSH.

NIOSH. 2006. NIOSH Hearing Loss Research Program: Details About Specific Studies Mentioned on Page 43 of the Evidence Package. Cincinnati, OH: NIOSH.

NIOSH. 2006. NIOSH Hearing Loss Research Program: Effectiveness of HPDs for Impulse Noise. Cincinnati, OH: NIOSH.

NIOSH. 2006. NIOSH Hearing Loss Research Program: Evaluation of the doseBusters USA Exposure Smart Protector. Cincinnati, OH: NIOSH.

NIOSH. 2006. NIOSH Hearing Loss Research Program: Evaluation Process for Intramural Research. Cincinnati, OH: NIOSH.

NIOSH. 2006. NIOSH Hearing Loss Research Program: FitCheck. Cincinnati, OH: NIOSH.

NIOSH. 2006. NIOSH Hearing Loss Research Program FTE FY97–FY05 (Excel spreadsheet). Cincinnati, OH: NIOSH.

NIOSH. 2006. NIOSH Hearing Loss Research Program: Funds Received from Other Agencies. Cincinnati, OH: NIOSH.

NIOSH. 2006. NIOSH Hearing Loss Research Program: HPDFit. Cincinnati, OH: NIOSH.

NIOSH. 2006. NIOSH Hearing Loss Research Program: Institute Strategic Planning Outline. Cincinnati, OH: NIOSH.

NIOSH. 2006. NIOSH Hearing Loss Research Program: Interaction with Stakeholders for Ford Study Mentioned on Page 54 of the EP. Cincinnati, OH: NIOSH.

NIOSH. 2006. NIOSH Hearing Loss Research Program: Intramural Projects and Budget Distribution, 1997–2005. Cincinnati, OH: NIOSH.

NIOSH. 2006. NIOSH Hearing Loss Research Program: NOES Database. Cincinnati, OH: NIOSH.

NIOSH. 2006. NIOSH Hearing Loss Research Program: OEP Project Officers (Scientific Program Administrators). Cincinnati, OH: NIOSH.

NIOSH. 2006. NIOSH Hearing Loss Research Program: Peer Review Process for Intramural Research. Cincinnati, OH: NIOSH.

NIOSH. 2006. NIOSH Hearing Loss Research Program: Questions from the Email Request of March 1, 2006, Related to RG2 and RG4. Cincinnati, OH: NIOSH.

NIOSH. 2006. NIOSH Hearing Loss Research Program: Research Staff Distribution by Organizational Unit. Cincinnati, OH: NIOSH.

NIOSH. 2006. NIOSH Hearing Loss Research Program: The Repackaging of NIOSH Hearing Loss Materials by Other Organizations. Cincinnati, OH: NIOSH.

NIOSH. 2006. NIOSH Hearing Loss Research Program Stakeholders. Cincinnati, OH: NIOSH.

NIOSH. 2006. NIOSH Hearing Loss Research Program: Summary of Extramural Project Plans (1996–2005). Cincinnati, OH: NIOSH.

NIOSH. 2006. NIOSH Hearing Loss Research Programs: Summary of Intramural Project Plans (1996–2005). Cincinnati, OH: NIOSH.

NIOSH. 2006. NIOSH Interactions with Selected Other Federal Agencies. Cincinnati, OH: NIOSH.

NIOSH. 2006. NIOSH NORA Hearing Loss Team White Paper. Cincinnati, OH: NIOSH.

NIOSH. 2006. NIOSH Program Portfolio. Cincinnati, OH: NIOSH.

NIOSH. 2006. NIOSH Strategic Plan Outline 2004–2009. Cincinnati, OH: NIOSH.

NIOSH. 2006. Pittsburgh Research Laboratory: Visitor Information. Pittsburgh, PA: NIOSH.

OMB (Office of Management and Budget). 2005. OMB Program Assessment Rating Tool (PART). Washington, DC.

Peterson JS, Kovalchik PG, Matetic RJ. 2005. A Sound Power Level Study of a Roof Bolter. Preprint No. 05-72, Society of Mining, Metallurgy and Exploration Annual Meeting, Salt Lake City, UT, February 28–March 2.

Rai A. 2005. Characterization of Noise and Design of Active Noise Control Technology in Longwall Mines. M.S. thesis. West Virginia University, Morgantown, WV.

Rai A, Luo Y, Slagley J, Peng SS, Guffey S. 2005. Survey and Experimental Studies on Engineering Control of Machine Noises in Longwall Mining Faces. Preprint 05-77, SME Annual Meeting, Salt Lake City, UT, February 28–March 2.

Schmitt JG (JGS Consulting). 2001. Evaluation of the Adequacy of the Anechoic Chamber at the University of Cincinnati for the Measurement and Reporting of Noise Emissions from Power Tools and Equipment: Initial Observations (slide set). Austin, TX: JGS Consulting.

Sinclair RC (NIOSH). 2006. FW: Mining Appropriations. E-mail to L Joellenbeck, Institute of Medicine. March 22.

Stephenson M. 2001. Protocol: Hearing Loss Prevention Program for Carpenters. Cincinnati, OH: NIOSH.

Stephenson CM. 2006. Research Goal 1: Contribute to the Development, Implementation, and Evaluation of Effective Hearing Loss Prevention Programs. Presentation to the Committee to Review the NIOSH Hearing Loss Research Program, Meeting I, January 5. Washington, DC.

Sweeney MH, Fosbroke D, Goldenhar LM, Jackson LL, Linch K, Lushniak BD, Merry C, Schneider S, Stephenson M. 2000. Health consequences of working in construction. In: Coble RJ, Hinze J, Haupt TC, eds. *Construction Safety and Health Management.* Upper Saddle River, NJ: Prentice-Hall. Pp. 211–234.

Tubbs RL. 2002. Memorandum: Close-out of HETA 95-0249; HETA 96-0007. Cincinnati, OH: NIOSH.

Tubbs RL, Kardous CA. 2006. Headset Noise Experienced by Medical Transcriptionists. Poster for NHCA Conference, Tampa, FL, February 17–19.

U.S. Congress. 1970. Occupational Safety and Health Act of 1970 (P.L. 91-596, abridged). Washington, DC: U.S. Congress.

Wade LV. 2006. Overview of NIOSH. Presentation to the Committee to Review the NIOSH Hearing Loss Research Program, Meeting I, January 5. Washington, DC.

D

Biographical Sketches of Committee Members

Bernard D. Goldstein, M.D. (*Chair*), is a professor in the Department of Environmental and Occupational Health and the former dean at the University of Pittsburgh Graduate School of Public Health. Previously he served as the director of the Environmental and Occupational Health Sciences Institute, a joint program of Rutgers, the State University of New Jersey, and the University of Medicine and Dentistry of New Jersey (UMDNJ)–Robert Wood Johnson Medical School. He was also principal investigator for the Consortium of Risk Evaluation with Stakeholder Participation (CRESP). Dr. Goldstein was assistant administrator for research and development, U.S. Environmental Protection Agency (EPA), 1983–1985. His past activities include serving as a member and chairman of the National Institutes of Health (NIH) Toxicology Study Section and EPA's Clean Air Scientific Advisory Committee; chair of the Institute of Medicine (IOM) Committee on the Role of the Physician in Occupational and Environmental Medicine, the National Research Council (NRC) Committees on Biomarkers in Environmental Health Research and Risk Assessment Methodology, and the Industry Panel of the World Health Organization (WHO) Commission on Health and Environment. He is a member of the IOM, where he has cochaired the section on Public Health, Biostatistics, and Epidemiology. He is a member and past president of the Society for Risk Analysis. He is a member and fellow of the American College of Environmental and Occupational Medicine, and a member of the Collegium Ramazzini, the Society for Occupational and Environmental Health, the Society of Toxicology, and the American Public Health Association. Dr. Goldstein is the past recipient of the Robert A. Kehoe Award of Merit of the American College of Occupational and Environmental Medicine. He received his medical degree from New York University.

Beth A. Cooper, M.S., is an acoustical engineer and manager of the Acoustical Testing Laboratory (ATL) at the NASA Glenn Research Center, where she provides noise control engineering support to help Glenn Research Center's science experiment payloads meet International Space Station hearing conservation goals. Under her direction, the ATL offers a comprehensive array of National Voluntary Laboratory Accreditation Program (NVLAP)-accredited testing, low-noise design, and educational services for the National Aeronautics and Space Administration (NASA) and external customers. The ATL also produces and distributes resources and training tools for use by hearing conservationists and noise control professionals. Ms. Cooper previously developed and managed Glenn Research Center's hearing conservation and community noise programs. She has managed the implementation of noise control projects for NASA's experimental facilities, as well as the design and construction of two major acoustical testing laboratories. Ms. Cooper is a registered professional engineer in the State of Ohio, a board-certified noise control engineer, and a certified occupational hearing conservationist. She has represented the Institute of Noise Control Engineering on the Council for Accreditation in Occupational Hearing Conservation and is a member of the study committee of the National Academy of Engineering project Technology for a Quieter America. Ms. Cooper is a frequent presenter on hearing conservation topics, with a special interest in presentation techniques and tools for effective hearing conservation training. She received her master's degree in acoustics from the Pennsylvania State University.

Susan E. Cozzens, Ph.D., is a professor of public policy at the Georgia Institute of Technology and director of its Technology Policy and Assessment Center. She is currently working on research in the fields of science, technology, and inequalities; and she continues to work internationally on developing methods for research assessment, as well as science and technology indicators. Before joining the faculty at the Georgia Institute of Technology, she was the director of the Office of Policy Support at the National Science Foundation (NSF). Dr. Cozzens has served as a consultant to numerous organizations, including the Office of Science and Technology Policy, NSF, the Office of Technology Assessment, the General Accounting Office, the National Cancer Institute, the National Institute on Aging, and NIH. She has served on several NRC and IOM committees, including Evaluation of the Sea Grant Program Review Process, Assessment of Centers of Excellence Programs at NIH, and Research Standards and Practices to Prevent the Destructive Application of Biotechnology. Dr. Cozzens is the past editor of *Science, Technology, & Human Values*, the journal of the Society for Social Studies of Science. She currently is the co-editor of *Research Evaluation*. She received her Ph.D. in sociology from Columbia University.

Karen J. Cruickshanks, Ph.D., is a professor in the Department of Ophthalmology and Visual Sciences as well as in the Department of Population Health Sciences at the University of Wisconsin School of Medicine and Public Health. She is the director of the Graduate Program in Population Health and the vice chair of the Department of Population Health Sciences. Her research interests are in the epidemiology of age-related sensory disorders, diabetes and its complications, and aging. She has written more than 100 articles on these topics and is the principal investigator for two major studies of the epidemiology of age-related hearing loss. Dr. Cruickshanks serves as frequent adviser or reviewer for the National Institute on Deafness and Other Communication Disorders (NIDCD) and as an ad hoc member of the NIH Neurological, Aging, and Musculoskeletal Epidemiology Study Section. She is a member of the Society for Epidemiological Research and the American Epidemiological Society. Dr. Cruickshanks previously served on the IOM Committee on Noise-Induced Hearing Loss and Tinnitus Associated with Military Service from World War II to the Present. She received her Ph.D. in epidemiology from the University of Pittsburgh.

Judy R. Dubno, Ph.D., is a professor in the Department of Otolaryngology–Head and Neck Surgery of the Medical University of South Carolina (MUSC). She is also a member of the MUSC Center for Advanced Imaging Research. Her research focuses on human auditory system function, with emphasis on the encoding of auditory information in simple sounds and speech, and how these abilities change in adverse listening conditions, with age, and with hearing loss. This research is currently funded by NIDCD of NIH. Dr. Dubno's other activities currently include serving as a member of the Executive Council of the Acoustical Society of America, the Tinnitus Research Consortium, and the Board of Directors of the Deafness Research Foundation. She previously served as a member of the National Deafness and Other Communication Disorders Advisory Council of the NIH, the NRC Committee on Hearing, Bioacoustics, and Biomechanics (CHABA), and the IOM Committee on Noise-Induced Hearing Loss and Tinnitus Associated with Military Service from World War II to the Present. She is a fellow of the Acoustical Society of America and the American Speech–Language–Hearing Association. Dr. Dubno holds a Ph.D. in speech/hearing science from the City University of New York Graduate School and University Center.

Dennis A. Giardino, M.S., is an acoustic consultant specializing in evaluation of the noise environments of industrial and mining facilities. Previously, Mr. Giardino served as chief of the Physical and Toxic Agents Division of the Mine Safety and Health Administration (MSHA). During his time as chief, he was responsible for providing technical support in protecting the health and safety of all miners in the United States with respect to harmful noise and vibration exposures, as well as editing and reviewing the current MSHA noise regulation for mining in the United States, overseeing noise investigation at mining facilities throughout the United States, and establishing and managing all of MSHA's primary acoustic laboratories. From 1973 to 1980, Mr. Giardino served as the chief of the Noise Branch of the U.S. Bureau of Mines, where he helped implement the then-new noise regulation for mining. He has published numerous research articles on noise associated with mining. Mr. Giardino received his master's in physics from the University of Pittsburgh.

Rena H. Glaser, M.A., retired as manager of medical surveillance for 3M Corporation in 2002, after nearly 30 years of service with the company in numerous capacities involving hearing conservation and occupational noise exposure. Ms. Glaser developed, managed, and led to international prominence the 3M hearing conservation program, with responsibility for more than 50 plants where more than 10,000 employees were enrolled in the program. Ms. Glaser is a member of the National Hearing Conservation Association (NHCA) and served as its president from 1984 to 1986. She received NHCA's Michael B. Threadgill Award for Outstanding Leadership and Service in 1992. Ms. Glaser has also been a member of American Speech–Language–Hearing Association and was awarded fellowship in 1990. Other professional memberships have included the American Auditory Society, the American Academy of Audiology, and the Acoustical Society of America, as well as several state professional organizations. She served as chair of the Council for Accreditation in Occupational Hearing Conservation, representing the American Speech–Language–Hearing Association. Ms. Glaser has been a frequent presenter and lecturer on occupational hearing conservation. She received her master's in audiology from the University of Illinois at Champaign–Urbana.

William W. Lang, Ph.D., currently serves as the president of the Noise Control Foundation and has held this position since 1975. Dr. Lang worked at the IBM Corporation from 1958 to 1992. While at IBM, he had corporate responsibility for the design of low-noise computers and business machines and for developing technical advances in the digital processing of acoustical signals. Dr. Lang has been involved extensively in international noise control engineering. He was a founding member of the Institute of Noise Control Engineering of the United States and cofounded the International Institute of Noise Control Engineering. Dr. Lang served as chair of the International Electrotechnical Commission–Technical Committee 29 on electroacoustics from 1975 to 1984, and he is currently serving as the convener of the International Organization for Standardization (ISO) Working Group on machinery noise emission standards. He is a member of the National Academy of Engineering and has served on several NRC committees, including CHABA. Dr. Lang has authored or coauthored more than 50 technical publications and has been the editor of two books. He is a fellow of the Institute of Electrical and Electronic Engineers, the Acoustical Society of America, the American Association for the Advancement of Science, the Audio Engineering Society, and the Institute of Acoustics. Dr. Lang holds a Ph.D. in physics and acoustics from Iowa State University.

Laura C. Leviton, Ph.D., is a senior program officer of the Robert Wood Johnson Foundation. She has overseen evaluations in most of the areas of focus for the foundation and now works primarily on initiatives in preventing childhood obesity and in serving vulnerable populations. Before joining the foundation she was a professor of public health at the University of Alabama at Birmingham and, before that, a member of the faculty of the University of Pittsburgh School of Public Health. Dr. Leviton is a leading writer on evaluation methods and practice, in particular for disease prevention. She was president of the American Evaluation Association in the year 2000, coauthored a leading evaluation text, and serves on several editorial boards for evaluation journals. She received the 1993 award from the American Psychological Association for Distinguished Contributions to Psychology in the Public Interest for her work in HIV prevention and health promotion at the workplace. She served on an IOM committee to evaluate preparedness for terrorist attacks and was a member of the Centers for Disease Control and Prevention's National Advisory Committee on HIV and STD (sexually transmitted disease) Prevention. She led a multihospital randomized trial to encourage the use of corticosteroid therapy in preterm infants and is a coinvestigator of a similar trial in conjunction with the Vermont–Oxford Network. She is coauthor of *Foundations of Program Evaluation: Theorists and Their Theories* and *Confronting Public Health Risks*. She received her Ph.D. in social psychology from the University of Kansas and postdoctoral training in evaluation research from Northwestern University.

Brenda L. Lonsbury-Martin, Ph.D., is a research professor in the Division of Otolaryngology–Head and Neck Surgery, Department of Surgery, at Loma Linda University School of Medicine. Her research interests include the early detection of hearing loss using otoacoustic emissions, the role of the cochlear efferent system in protecting the ear from noise damage, mechanisms of noise- and drug-induced hearing loss, and cochlear plasticity. Dr. Lonsbury-Martin has been developing special-purpose protocols using otoacoustic emissions to evaluate, screen, and monitor the functional status of the hearing portion of the inner ear over the past 20 years. She is a fellow of the Acoustical Society of America and the American Academy of Otolaryngology–Head and Neck Surgery (AAOHNS), and she is a member of the American Academy of Audiology, the American Auditory Society (AAS), the American Speech–Language–Hearing Association, the Association for Research in Otolaryngology, and the Society for Neuroscience. Dr. Lonsbury-Martin is an associate editor of *Physiological Acoustics/Peripheral Ear* for the *Journal of the Acoustical Society of America* and a member of the editorial boards of *Hearing Research* and the *Journal of the American Academy of Audiology*. She also serves on the study section review panels of several private foundations, including AAOHNS and the Tinnitus Research Consortium, as well as serving on the AAS Board of Directors. Dr. Lonsbury-Martin received her Ph.D. in neuroscience and physiology from Oregon Health and Science University and completed postdoctoral fellowship training in psychobiology and physiology and biophysics at the University of California, Irvine, and the University of Washington, respectively.

Michael A. Silverstein, M.D., M.P.H., is a clinical professor in the Department of Environmental and Occupational Health Sciences at the University of Washington School of Public Health and Community Medicine. He previously worked for the State of Washington, serving as the assistant director for industrial safety and health in the Department of Labor and Industries and as the state health officer in the Department of Health. He spent 2 years as the director of policy for the Occupational Safety and Health Administration in the U.S. Department of Labor and 15 years as the assistant director of health and safety at the United Automobile Workers International Union. Dr. Silverstein recently served as the chair of the Occupational Health and Safety Section of the American Public Health Association. He is a fellow of the American College of Occupational and Environmental Medicine. Dr. Silverstein has previously served on several NRC committees, including the health and safety needs of older workers and the health and safety implications of child labor. He has an M.D. from Stanford University School of Medicine and an M.P.H. from the University of Michigan School of Public Health and is board certified in occupational medicine.

FRAMEWORK COMMITTEE LIAISON

Franklin E. Mirer, Ph.D., is the director of the Health and Safety Department for the United Automobile, Aerospace and Agricultural Implement Workers of America (UAW). His primary scientific interest is exposure and risk assessment in the occupational environment. Dr. Mirer has served on several National Academies committees, including Institutional Means for Risk Assessment, Risk Assessment Methodology, Review of the Health Effects Institute, and currently serves on the Review of NIOSH Research Programs. He has testified before House and Senate committees on occupational safety and health matters. Dr. Mirer was inducted into the National Safety Council's Health and Safety Hall of Fame and is a fellow of the Collegium Ramazzini and the American Industrial Hygiene Association. He holds appointments as an adjunct professor at the University of Michigan School of Public Health, adjunct associate professor at the Mt. Sinai School of Medicine, and visiting lecturer at the Harvard School of Public Health. He has a Ph.D. in physical organic chemistry from Harvard University and is a toxicologist and certified industrial hygienist.